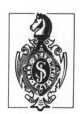

Richard Godwin-Austen · John Bendall

The Neurology
of the Elderly

Springer-Verlag
London Berlin Heidelberg New York
Paris Tokyo Hong Kong

Richard Godwin-Austen MD, FRCP
Consultant Neurologist, Nottingham University and Derby Hospitals, Department
of Neurology, University Hospital, Queen's Medical Centre, Nottingham NG7 2UH

John Bendall BSc, DM, FRCP
Senior Lecturer/Consultant Physician in Health Care of the Elderly, University
Hospital, Queen's Medical Centre, Nottingham NG7 2UH

ISBN 3-540-19593-9   Springer-Verlag Berlin Heidelberg New York
ISBN 0-387-19593-9   Springer-Verlag New York Berlin Heidelberg

British Library Cataloguing in Publication Data
Godwin-Austen, Richard
The neurology of the elderly.
1. Old persons. Nervous system. Diseases
I. Title II. Bendall, John
618.97
ISBN 3-540-19593-9

Library of Congress Cataloging-in-Publication Data
Godwin-Austen, R. B.
The neurology of the elderly/Richard Godwin-Austen and John Bendall.
p.   cm. Includes bibliographical references.
ISBN 0-387-19593-9
1. Geriatric neurology. I. Bendall, John, 1943–   . II. Title.
[DNLM: 1. Nervous System Diseases—in old age. 2. Neurologic
Manifestations—in old age. WL   100 G657n]
RC346.G62   1990   618.97′68—dc20   DNLM/DLC
for Library of Congress   89-26156
                                                                CIP

Filmset by Macmillan India Ltd, Bangalore 560 025
Printed by The Bath Press, Avon, UK.
2128/3916-543210   Printed on acid-free paper

Do not cast me away when I am old;
do not forsake me when my strength is gone

Psalms 71:9

Acknowledgements

We would like to acknowledge with gratitude the comments and help we received from Tony Blake and Roy Boyd.

Mrs Jene Webster was responsible for the manuscript and her assistance is gratefully acknowledged.

Preface

Traditional methods in the clinical practice of neurology have dominated clinical teaching in this specialty for about 100 years. Essentially these methods involve meticulous attention to detail and the recording of clinical facts. Thus the clinical history must be recorded chronologically, preferably in the patient's own words, and followed by a carefully structured examination of the nervous system set out in such a way as to allow the precise localisation of the lesion or system involved. Clinical neurology taught and practised in this way has bred generations of neurologists throughout the world and raised the standards in the specialty to a level where clinical skills are probably unexcelled in any other specialty. With increasing availability and reliance upon non-invasive imaging techniques, the need for these skills in large areas of neurological practice has diminished. But perhaps more importantly, the classical clinical methods in neurology were developed when the elderly population was much smaller and when the specialty of geriatrics did not exist. As a result, much of the methodology is irrelevant or unreliable in the elderly population and the student of geriatrics will frequently find himself searching in vain in the textbooks of neurology for help in assessing an elderly patient with an atypical presentation (for example disturbance of balance or recurrent confusional episodes) of some common neurological disorder.

Where a structural abnormality of the central nervous system may account for the symptoms or signs in an old person, computed tomography (CT) or magnetic resonance imaging will frequently lead to rapid and accurate assessment of the patient's therapeutic needs and prognosis. But there are many situations where such structural disorder does not enter the differential diagnosis, or where the CT scan is normal. In these cases the clinician is forced to exercise his clinical skills but may find that the classical methods of detailed history-taking and examination fail to resolve the problem.

This book is written with this dilemma in mind. The text is "problem-orientated", so that some of the commonest problems in the elderly are discussed in terms of clinical evaluation, investigation and differential diagnosis and management. History-taking–on which so much depends in the neurological assessment of the younger patient–is frequently limited in scope in the elderly by forgetfulness, confusion or nervousness in a frail individual. Similarly, physical signs in the old may be less reliable than in the young. Apparent wasting of the hands, absent reflexes and apparent sensory disturbances are frequently extremely difficult to evaluate even by the most experienced clinician. The first chapter of this book is devoted to consideration of these problems.

Henry Miller once said "the chief value of a neurologist is to prevent the over-investigation of the neurological patient". Over-investigation is wasteful, distressing and time-consuming to the patient; and with invasive investigations carries significant risk for the elderly as well as causing them discomfort. It is, therefore, even more important in the old than it is in the young to avoid unnecessary investigations and always to bear in mind the scope for therapeutic intervention–particularly surgery. The judicious use of scanning and other investigation techniques in the old provides the material for the second chapter of this book.

The aim has been to provide a short text suitable for use by the practising geriatrician or trainee neurologist or geriatrician and also by the general physician and general practitioner.

This is a practical text which does not hope to be comprehensive in its consideration of diseases likely to afflict the old. No detailed consideration is given, for example, to cerebral vascular disease–there are many comprehensive texts devoted to this subject. It is not the aim of this book to include matters such as the detailed assessment of a patient for neurosurgery. Similarly neuropathology, neurochemistry and neurophysiology have not been included in any detail but only where an understanding of these subjects is essential to the clinical management of the patient.

Finally rehabilitation, and social services occupy a vital place in the treatment of neurological disturbances in the old. These paramedical specialties have been referred to only briefly and no attempt has been made to consider their organisation or methodology in any detail.

Nottingham   Richard Godwin-Austen
May 1989   John Bendall

Contents

1 The Neurological Examination of The Elderly Patient   1

History-taking   2
The General Examination   5
Temperature   7
Blood Pressure   8
Aids, Appliances and Chairs   8
The Neurological Examination   8

2 The Investigation of the Elderly Patient 13

Lumbar Puncture 15
Computed Tomography (CT) Scan 17
Electroencephalography (EEG) 18
Electromyography (EMG) and Nerve Conduction
    Velocity (NCV) 20
Evoked Potential Recording 21
Myelography 21
Angiography 22
Magnetic Resonance Imaging (MRI) 23

3 "Confusion" and Dementia 25

History 26
Examination 28
    Tests of Memory 29
    Tests of Language Function 30
    Visuo-spatial Disorientation 30
    Physical Examination 31
Acute and Subacute Organic Brain Syndromes 32
    Confusional States due to Drugs 34
    Nocturnal Behavioural Disturbance 34
    Nutritional and Toxic Confusional States 35

Dementia: Chronic Organic Brain Syndromes   36
   Senile Dementia of the Alzheimer Type (SDAT)   36
   The Vascular (Arteriosclerotic or Multi-infarct)
   Dementias   37
   "Reversible Dementias"   39
   Subcortical Dementia   40
Parkinson's Disease and Dementia   40
Dementia of Frontal Type   41
Normal Pressure Hydrocephalus   41
Pseudodementia   41

4 Disturbances of Gait and Balance, and Falls   43

Maintenance of Posture and the Effects of Age and
Age-related Disease   44
   Sensory   44
   Motor   46
   Musculo-skeletal Changes   47
Neuropathies   48
Subacute Combined Degeneration of the Cord   48
Gait Dyspraxia   49
   Treatment   51

5 Headache and Facial Neuralgia   53

Headache   54
   Extracranial Headache   54
   Intracranial Headache   58
   Psychogenic Headache   61
Facial Neuralgia   62
   Trigeminal Neuralgia   62
   Post-herpetic Neuralgia   64
   Migrainous Syndromes   64
   Atypical Facial Pain   64

6 Some Visual Problems   67

Episodic Visual Disturbance   68
   Amaurosis fugax   68
   Migraine   69
   Epilepsy   70
Persistent and Progressive Visual Disturbance   71
   Prechiasmal (and Retrobulbar) Lesions   71
   Retrochiasmal Lesions   72
Double Vision   72
Visual Hallucinations and Disorders of Visual Perception .   75

7 Incontinence 77

Urinary Incontinence 78
   Normal Control of the Bladder 78
   The Effect of Ageing 79
   History of Urinary Incontinence 79
   Examination and Investigation 80
   The Causes of Urinary Incontinence 81
Faecal Incontinence 83
   Normal Control of Defaecation 84
   History of Faecal Incontinence 85
   Examination 85
Conclusion 86

8 Parkinsonism and Abnormal Movement Disorders 87

The Presenting Symptoms and Signs of Parkinsonism 88
The Examination of the Patient with Parkinsonism 90
   The Tremor 90
   Hypokinesia 91
   Rigidity 91
Other Signs in Parkinsonism 92
   Disorders of Gait 92
   Disorders of Higher Mental Function 93
   Autonomic Function 93
   Eye Signs 94
Assessment 94
Course 94
Parkinson's Disease and Senile Parkinsonism 95
   Management 96
Abnormal Movement Disorders: Dystonias 98
   Dystonia 98
   Facial Dyskinesia 99
   Dystonic Dysarthria 99

9 Attacks of Loss of Consciousness and Disturbance of Memory 101

Attacks of Loss of Consciousness 101
   History, Examination and Investigation 103
   Epilepsy 104
   Cardiac Dysrrhythmias 105
   Postural Hypotension 106
   Cough and Micturition Syncope 106
   "Drop Attacks" 106
   Vertebro-basilar Ischaemia 107
   Post-stroke "Narcolepsy" and Drowsiness 107
   Hypothermia 108

Amnesic States 108
Wernicke's Encephalopathy and Korsakoff's Psychosis . 109
Transient Global Amnesia 110
Amnesia in Diffuse Cerebral Disorder 111

10 Loss of Use in the Upper Limb 113

The History 114
The Examination 114
The Signs 115
"Numbness" 119
Abnormal Involuntary Movements 123
Tremor 123
Choreo-athetosis 123
Dystonia 124
Dyspraxia 124

**11 Neurological Presentations of General Medical
Disorders** 127

Diabetesm Mellitus 127
Hypoglycaemia 129
Thyroid Disease 130
Disorders of Water and Mineral Metabolism 132
Disorders of Calcium Metabolism 133
Alcohol and Alcoholism 135
Nutritional and other Vitamin Deficiencies 138
Neuropsychiatric Manifestations of Malignant Disease . . 139
Herpes Zoster 140
Myeloma and Dysproteinaemias 141
Drugs 141

References and Further Reading 143

Subject Index 144

1 The Neurological Examination of the Elderly Patient

In medical practice the elderly form a heterogeneous group so that those aged between 65 and 75 years are generally fit and active while those over 75 years (the very elderly) are more likely to suffer multiple diseases, which present atypically and lead to progressive disability and dependence. This book is concerned mainly with the neurology of the very elderly in whom common neurological disorders often present in a non-specific way and in whom the signs and symptoms of neurological disease may be difficult to elicit or assess. Clinical findings which may be caused by neurological disease may also be due to other conditions, the patient thus requiring detailed assessment in order to make a definitive diagnosis. In patients over 75 years of age neurological disease commonly co-exists with other conditions which may modify symptoms and signs: for example the presenting disease may be a stroke, but the patient may also have arthritis and dementia, both of which may alter the patient's response to and recovery from the stroke. It must also be remembered that the subsequent complication rate from all medical conditions is much higher in the very elderly than in younger people.

In geriatric practice atypical or non-specific presentation of common conditions is the norm. These presentations include falls, immobility, incontinence, confusion, acute "acopia" (relatives or other carers being unable to cope) and hypothermia, the last often being secondary to other illnesses which may be occult. The aged patient's clinical state may be compounded by iatrogenic illness due to multiple therapy for multiple diseases and to alterations in pharmacokinetics (what the body does to drugs in relation to their absorption, distribution and excretion) and pharmacodynamics (what drugs do to the body). It is in this context that the neurological examination of the elderly must be considered.

Much of what applies to the examination of younger individuals applies equally to the elderly, but multiple diseases and non-specific presentation may create particular problems. A full history and physical examination is even more essential than in the young but it is not proposed to discuss these aspects in detail in this book. This chapter will concentrate on the particular difficulties and pitfalls in history-taking and examination of the elderly, including factors related to the functional assessment of the patient and the initial planning of rehabilitation. The majority of the very elderly are women and the feminine gender is therefore used throughout unless points specific to male patients are being discussed.

History-taking

History-taking can be a prolonged process. The patient should be as comfortable as possible and distractions reduced to a minimum. She must be able to see the interviewer's face so the room should be well lit: this is particularly important if she is deaf, so that she is able to lip-read. Observation of the patient during spontaneous activity is of special importance in assessing the neurological state and often provides more information than a prolonged neurological examination.

It is equally important to listen carefully to what the patient says; it is often a chance remark that gives the clue as to what is going on.

Case 1.1
An 80-year-old male reported having "funny turns", during which he became at first faint and shortly afterwards unconscious for a period varying from a few seconds up to 20 minutes. The attacks, occurring three or four times a week, were always preceded by a few seconds of palpitations in the chest, and an initial diagnosis of a cardiac dysrrhythmia was made. By chance the patient remarked that on several occasions he had looked at his chest at the onset of these attacks and had observed that he could "even see my chest wall twitching, the palpitations were so strong"; he had drawn his wife's attention to this phenomenon. His wife confirmed the observation, and added that the twitching seemed to spread from his chest upwards into the left side of his neck and left arm and afterwards down into the left leg. Eventually his whole body was involved in what now was clearly a Jacksonian fit and he would be incontinent. A 24-h ECG suggested that the fits were precipitated by a supraventricular tachycardia resulting in decreased cerebral perfusion. At first treatment with verapamil controlled both the tachycardia and the fits, but when, 2 years later, the "funny turns" recurred in the absence of any tachycardia, the patient's previous chance comment about his twitching chest and the resulting description by his wife of a Jacksonian fit, led to his successful treatment with phenytoin.

Slowness of verbal response to questions should not necessarily be taken as evidence of mental impairment; the elderly usually answer questions more slowly than the young and it is, therefore, essential to take time in history-taking. Depression, myxoedema and Parkinson's disease may also be responsible for a slow response. High-tone deafness is common in old age and the interviewer should speak to the patient in a low-pitched voice; failure to appreciate that she may be deaf can lead to an incorrect diagnosis of dementia.

If she has a hearing aid, make sure that it is working properly and in use for the interview; failing this, many hospital wards and clinics now have speech amplifiers for use with the deaf.

In order to form some idea of whether the patient's history is accurate it is important, early in the interview, to try to assess her mental function. Bear in mind, however, that if a formal assessment of memory is carried out too early in the consultation a mentally normal patient may be offended by being asked apparently simple questions which make her feel that she is being treated as "an idiot". Such a formal assessment should, therefore, only be carried out when a good rapport has been established. Early in the interview clues of memory loss should be sought in inconsistencies in the patient's replies to other questions and in comments spontaneously made; for example, referring to deceased relatives as if they were still alive, or claims to be doing all the housework when it is already known that she is receiving extensive support from social service agencies or from her family, or that her home is in a neglected state.

Collateral evidence from the patient's relatives, neighbours, friends, home help, social workers and general practitioner may be essential in obtaining an accurate picture of what has been happening to her. An independent history is essential when the patient is demented, amnesic or dysphasic, has impairment of consciousness, or is distracted by pain or other symptoms. Some such information may be contained in the referral letter, or pressed on the doctor, unsolicited, by anxious relatives prior to the consultation. This information should not always be taken at face value. Often relatives (and the patient) will claim that "she has a marvellous memory" or "she's as clear as a bell": these remarks may be based on the patient's memory for events long past which is often well preserved in the early stages of dementia. Specific questions about current daily activities and safety are useful; does she leave the gas unlit, or burn pots and pans on the stove? Any elderly patient whose memory shows evidence from the history of possible impairment should have a simple test of mental function towards the end of the initial interview, the most commonly used test being the Abbreviated Mental Test. This test and other aspects of the assessment of cognitive function are discussed in detail in Chapter 3. Bear in mind that a good social facade linked with confabulation can deceive even the most wary into a false assessment.

Patients who have normal memory may, even so, be totally unrealistic about their capabilities. Denial of disability is a common response and probably represents a defence against having to take unpalatable decisions or having to "climb down", for example when strongly held views such as "I'll never go into an old folks' home" have been espoused. Again corroboration from others is helpful.

The time course of events in the recent illness and the nature and timing of previous episodes or "funny turns" gives valuable information about likely aetiology. Sudden deterioration in health is associated with an acute event (for example, myocardial infarction, pulmonary embolus, stroke or infection); long-term deterioration is due to chronic illnesses such as arthritis, recurrent small strokes, dementia, Parkinson's disease and other degenerative conditions. It is important to ask specifically whether the presenting symptom, including falls, incontinence, confusion or "acopia", is of recent onset or is long-standing and perhaps of increasing severity.

Elderly patients and their relatives may consider that all is well – a perception sometimes wrongly based on low expectations of what the elderly are like and can do. Specific questions about washing, dressing, cooking, toiletting and shopping give much more information about what the patient is really like. Most elderly individuals are independent in these activities. Other markers of dependency include the amount of support in the form of home help, meals on wheels, district nurse, family involvement and attendance at day centres and day hospitals that is required.

Questions about functional ability prior to the index illness are useful not only in assessing the time course of the condition, but also in determining the level of recovery that might be expected following treatment and rehabilitation. Someone who was totally independent prior to the illness has a better chance of subsequently achieving functional independence than someone with chronic disability. An accurate review of previous independence or dependence allows realistic goals to be set from the beginning of rehabilitation.

Iatrogenic illness has already been mentioned. It is essential to check very carefully which drugs the patient is taking: the GP may only mention one or two (usually the ones most recently prescribed) and may assume that this is all the patient takes. Elderly patients, however, frequently hoard drugs from previous episodes of illness and use the drugs subsequently when they feel it is appropriate, whether it is or not. Try to find out which drugs the patient has at home: showing them to her may prompt a more accurate picture of current medication.

Case 1.2
An 82-year-old female was admitted with a history of falling. She described falls occurring just after she got out of bed or stood up from a chair. The falls which had been going on for a fortnight were accompanied by a sensation of dizziness and faintness. If she felt these sensations coming on and was able to sit down quickly they rapidly disappeared. She had adopted a strategy of getting up very slowly out of bed in the mornings, first sitting on the edge of the bed for about fifteen minutes whilst she had a cup of tea from her "Teasmaid". The main physical finding was a postural fall in blood pressure from 180/90 in the lying position, to 140/70 on standing. The patient denied taking medication prior to admission and her GP had specifically stated that she was on no medication. When the patient's daughter was asked to bring in to the ward any tablets in her mother's house, a bottle of bendrofluazide tablets appeared. When shown these tablets the patient remembered that she had been taking the tablets for several weeks. She had originally been given the diuretic for heart failure and had probably taken them rather erratically though in sufficient quantities to render her symptom-free. When, three years later, she developed swelling of her legs unassociated with any dyspnoea, and probably due to venous incompetence, she remembered the "water tablets" and started taking them again, thus precipitating postural hypotension. This disorder settled spontaneously during a 10-day period in hospital.

Certain symptoms, possibly indicating neurological disorder, may be difficult to evaluate in the elderly. Pain is often ill-defined; the patient may use terms such as "discomfort", "numbness" or "weakness" to indicate true pain, irritation of the skin, hyperaesthesia, tingling or even loss of cutaneous sensation. Careful questioning is required to clarify what is meant. In some cases, for example the prodromal pain of *Herpes zoster*, the fact that the symptom occurs within an anatomically defined area (nerve root distribution) will suggest possible pathological processes. In other patients the way in which factors such as food, rest, position, movement or drugs affect the "numbness" may indicate the cause. Dizziness is a term that can cover a multitude of feelings; it can refer to unsteadiness on walking, strange sensations in the head, tinnitus, vertigo, headache, feelings of tightness in the head, nausea, borborigmi, or even abdominal pain. Unsteadiness is another term similarly ill-defined. No such term should be taken at face value but should be carefully probed, bearing in mind that these non-specific terms sometimes reflect underlying psychological abnormality (for example, neuroticism), or variation in perception of symptoms due to upbringing, culture and race.

Patients with weakness from hemi- or para-plegia are best assessed for severity of their symptoms by recording the degree of functional disability they suffer. How far can they walk? Can they climb stairs? Can they get out of a bath? When were they last able to walk to the Post Office, etc? Similar questions apply in patients with Parkinson's disease where the drug treatment advised may depend on the severity and rate of progression of the symptoms.

The General Examination

Most of what applies in the general examination of younger patients applies equally to the elderly. Several features are, however, of particular significance in the elderly and it is to these that the remainder of this chapter is devoted.

The condition of the patient's home indicates both her abilities over a period of time and the level and effectiveness of support being provided. The state of her attire and general level of cleanliness are also useful indicators.

Abnormalities of sensation and communication often lead to isolation. Hearing loss may be obvious, but lesser degrees of impairment may be assessed during history-taking by varying the volume with which questions are asked. Wax in the external auditory meatus is unlikely to impair hearing significantly in someone with otherwise normal function but, in a patient who has an underlying hearing loss, wax may lead to unnecessary further reduction. Hearing aids are often not worn even when prescribed: check that the aid is working. Patients frequently do not realise that hearing aids are primarily aimed at improving "one-to-one" communication, and are of no real benefit in crowded noisy places. Aids are often left on continuously and the batteries quickly run down, so it is important to check that the patient knows how to use the aid.

If the patient has poor vision make sure that her spectacles are clean. Dirty lenses are a common problem in immobile patients. Poor vision should be assessed by ophthalmoscopy and by recording the visual fields to confrontation. Visual acuity should be measured using the Snellen chart with the patient wearing distance spectacles if they are available. If her glasses are not available, a visual acuity measurement with the patient reading the chart through a pin-hole will distinguish the patient with refractory error from the patient with some other defect causing loss of acuity.

Many neurological disorders produce abnormalities of speech. In the elderly, however, speech may be unclear due to the effect of ageing processes on speech mechanisms, and due to problems with dentition, both original and prosthetic. In the very elderly, speech is commonly slower than in the young, of higher pitch and lower volume. In patients with dentures the "portcullis" sign (the top denture falling on to the lower when the mouth is opened) may be due to poor fitting but developing *de novo* may be seen in cases of dehydration, or stroke leading to loss of tone in the buccal musculature. Oro-facial-dyskinesia or dystonic dysarthria may affect speech (See Chap. 8). Other extrapyramidal disorders, for example, Parkinson's disease may also lead to dysarthria.

Examination of the feet is important not only in respect of specific neurological signs but also for evidence of other pathology which may in itself adversely affect walking and gait, or which may do so when combined with a neurological disorder. Thus, patients who have difficulty in bending, have clumsy hands or who have poor vision are likely to be unable to cut their toe nails, which in turn commonly leads to pain on walking or even immobility. In grossly neglected patients onychogryphosis may develop, requiring expert chiropody.

Well-fitting footwear is important for good mobility. Poorly-fitting slippers or shoes may be hazardous and replacement with appropriate shoes (rather than slippers) may result in a significant improvement in walking. Sometimes the pattern of wear on the sole of the shoes gives a clue to underlying pathology; a patient with foot-drop due to a minor stroke may have increased wear over the outer anterior aspect of the sole on the affected side, whereas a patient with Parkinson's disease may have wear over the central or anterior part of the soles of both shoes due to shuffling gait.

The many skin diseases found in the elderly are outside the remit of the present text: the skin is, however, of major importance in elderly patients with severe neurological disease and immobility, because of the propensity to develop pressure sores. Particular attention must be given to skin over bony prominences (the "pressure areas"). Reddening may be a warning of undue pressure, but if associated with surrounding induration indicates necrosis of subcutaneous tissues. The "iceberg" phenomenon may be found – a small superficial area of necrosis or ulceration with a much larger surrounding area of induration, which is easily overlooked, but which indicates the true extent of necrotic tissue. When such ulcers get bigger causing concern to nursing staff who view this enlargement as a failure of nursing care, reassurance should be given that what is happening is inevitable as part of the evolution of the lesion, revealing its true extent.

Table 1.1. Scoring system to determine risk of developing pressure sores

Physical state		Mental state		Activity		Mobility		Incontinence	
Good	4	Alert	4	Ambulant	4	Full	4	None (include catheterised patients)	4
Fair	3	Apathetic	3	Walk with help	3	Slightly limited	3	Occasional	3
Poor	2	Confused	2	Chairfast	2	Very limited	2	Usually urine (include doubly incontinent but catheterised patients)	2
Very	1	Stuporous	1	Bedfast	1	Immobile	1	Doubly	1

A score of 14 points or below indicates a liability of subsequently developing pressure sores; 12 points or fewer indicate the risk to be very great. (Derived from Norton, McLaren and Exton-Smith 1962).

Pressure sores are an immediate possibility in any patient developing paralysis of the lower limbs, particularly if there is any associated loss of cutaneous sensation. The prevention of pressure sores is vital as they represent a source of sepsis and pain, are a metabolic drain, and a hindrance to rehabilitation, particularly when sited over the heels. A high level of awareness by the nursing staff in hospital or the family at home of the possibility of the development of pressure sores is essential in the management of the immobile patient, but this can be facilitated by use of a risk-scoring system of the type developed by Norton, McLaren and Exton-Smith (1962) (Table 1.1).

Temperature

A single measurement of body temperature may show the patient to be pyrexial (temperature above 37.5°C) or hypothermic (temperature below 35°C) at a particular point in time, but often in the elderly the shape of the temperature curve gives more information than a single reading; thus a patient may be ill with a chest infection with the body temperature remaining in the normal range, but the temperature chart usually shows a rise of the patient's temperature within the normal range. Hypothermia is of particular importance: it has a high mortality but is often missed, either from failure to take the patient's temperature, or because the measurement is made with a thermometer which is not a low-reading one; the temperature of the elderly should always be taken, if possible rectally, with a thermometer reading down to at least 30°C. From the neurological point of view, hypothermia is important as a cause of drowsiness or, in extreme cases, coma.

Blood Pressure

High blood pressure is usually not of immediate concern in an elderly patient. The evidence that treatment of hypertension in the very elderly is of benefit is poor and indeed recent experimental evidence indicates that, in over 80-yr-olds, high blood pressure may even be associated with increased survival. Stroke may be associated with elevated blood pressure, but this usually settles spontaneously over the course of a few days. Inappropriate use of antihypertensive agents may lead to postural hypotension (see below) or in extreme cases to falls in cerebral blood flow sufficient to cause or exacerbate the stroke. In previously hypertensive elderly patients even reduction of blood pressure to "normal" levels may be dangerous.

Postural hypotension is more important in the elderly than hypertension. It is arbitrarily defined as a fall in systolic blood pressure of more than 20-mm Hg when the patient rises from the lying to the standing position. The condition may be found incidentally, but is often of importance in leading to falls, dizziness and faintness, all of which will be discussed in greater detail later. In the early stages of postural hypotension the fall in blood pressure may only be detectable when the patient first rises in the morning, when the circulating blood volume is at its lowest; blood pressure recordings at this time of day are, therefore, particularly useful in detecting the condition.

Aids, Appliances and Chairs

Information about aids, appliances and chairs is essential in assessing what the patient has been able to do at home and how she did it, and also in deciding whether her disability was helped or hindered by the aids and appliances available to her. When the patient is seen at home the aids and appliances may be examined to determine their suitability, safety and any faults which may be present. If the patient is first seen in hospital, it may be necessary for the aid to be brought to the hospital, or for it to be examined at home by the occupational therapist near the time of discharge. Aids, appliances and chairs will not be discussed in detail in this book and the reader is recommended to read the excellent series of articles on the subject recently published in the British Medical Journal (Mulley 1989).

The Neurological Examination

The principles of neurological examination which apply to young patients apply equally to the elderly. But in the elderly eliciting abnormal signs and interpreting them is often much more difficult. The patient may not be able to co-operate fully because of confusion or dementia, so that sensory testing becomes unreliable. In an elderly person the neurological examination can be very tiring and her concentration may be lost; if this seems to be happening it is best to discontinue and to test again when the patient is rested. It may be necessary to return to the patient several times before one can be confident of findings that depend on her co-operation. The doctor inexperienced in examining the elderly can find himself faced with a number of signs which do not "hang together" in terms of "classical neurology" and consequently may fail to see the wood for the trees. Minor changes in signs are often important in diagnosis. For example, slight changes in symmetry of reflexes or tone on the two sides of the body may indicate new or progressing pathology. Detailed serial records must, therefore, be kept so that they can be referred back to subsequently.

No examination of an elderly patient is complete without seeing her walk. The pattern of walking may be affected by many factors – articular, muscular and neurological. Characteristic gaits are seen in conditions such as stroke, Parkinson's disease and cerebellar disorders. Some neurological signs seem to be consistently altered in the elderly. Impairment of conjugate upward gaze is commonly seen in the very elderly, where it has little or no significance. This contrasts with the younger patient where impairment of conjugate upward gaze may indicate hydrocephalus or an upper brainstem disorder. Other disorders of eye movement in the elderly have the same significance as they do in the young. The pupils are commonly small and dilate poorly to light; they may also be irregular as a result of previous iritis or, as is sometimes thought, due to age-related changes. The pupillary changes make fundoscopy difficult and it is sometimes necessary to dilate the pupil with a mydriatic to obtain a satisfactory view; even if dilatation is achieved the fundus may still be obscured by cataracts.

It is often difficult to get the patient to relax for testing muscle tone. The ankle jerks are often absent or reduced in otherwise normal elderly people. Sensory testing may be particularly difficult in the elderly. Vibration sense is commonly lost below the knees and in most cases this loss is of no significance; if, however, it is combined with loss of joint position sense it is more likely to indicate underlying pathology, though joint position sense can be extremely difficult to test, particularly if the patient has hallux valgus or arthritic toes, or has difficulty in co-operating with the test as a result of deafness or dementia. In the lower limbs testing for cutaneous sensation – both light touch and pinpoint–blunt discrimination – may be difficult. This is particularly so in the presence of oedema which (by stretching the skin and hence separating cutaneous sensory receptors) can lead to a reduction in both modalities. Oedema may also cause the leg to be painful and in some patients this may lead to inconsistent responses to cutaneous stimuli.

Tendon reflexes in the arms are often found to be brisk in older patients in the absence of other neurological signs. In some, this may be due to anxiety or to metabolic abnormality, most commonly dehydration due to other major illness. With reassurance and treatment of dehydration the reflexes usually return to normal, but in a proportion of patients they persist, giving rise to the suspicion that there is some underlying neurological disorder, probably diffuse vascular disease. This suspicion is heightened if the patient also has evidence of cognitive impairment, even if the latter does not show the typical step-wise pattern of progression of multi-infarct dementia. In patients thought to have had minor strokes the usually tested tendon reflexes may be inconclusive and difficult to compare. Finger jerks may be a more sensitive indicator. The pectoralis major tendon reflex, is tested for by getting the patient to sit up with the hands lightly resting on the hips, the examiner standing behind the patient placing his hand over the lower edge of the muscle and tapping the back of his hand with the tendon hammer. It may be useful in that the strength of contraction of the muscle can be felt as much as seen, and consequently be easier to compare with the other side.

The assessment of muscle wasting in the hands and forearms can be difficult, particularly in men and especially in extreme old age. Atrophic changes in the skin, with loss of subcutaneous tissue, may give appearances suggestive of small muscle wasting. If there are fasciculations at rest, if there is asymmetry between the hands, if there is focal wasting affecting thenar muscles but not the interossei (or vice versa) and, finally, if there is demonstrable weakness, then the wasting is probably real. But in the absence of these features, doubtful "wasting" is probably within normal limits.

The triceps jerks are quite often absent in the elderly, presumably from spondylotic changes in the neck; this abnormality is rarely associated with symptoms.

Other important features in the examination of the arms are discussed in Chapter 10.

Plantar reflexes can be difficult to elicit and to assess. The withdrawal response is common, but can sometimes be suppressed by repeating the test whilst getting the patient to lock her fingers together and "pull hard apart", or by getting the patient to squeeze something tightly in her hands. If one plantar shows a withdrawal or equivocal response then the other should do so as well, and a difference between the two suggests an underlying neurological abnormality.

Certain so-called "primitive reflexes" may be present, particularly in demented patients or in those with extensive cerebro-vascular disease. The palmo-mental reflex is elicited by stroking the finger across the patient's palm and observing contraction of the muscles over the chin on the same side. The grasp reflex is tested in the same way and is present if the patient involuntarily grasps the examiner's finger when it is placed against the palm of the patient's hands. The rooting reflex is elicited by stroking the patient's face on the cheek at the level of the mouth and observing whether her mouth twitches towards the stroked side. The presence of these reflexes is an indication of extensive brain disease affecting particularly the frontal lobe.

Co-ordination testing may be affected by arthritis which can limit joint movement, and muscle power may be impossible to assess in the presence of pain and stiffness in a joint, especially the shoulder or hip.

Time spent looking for fasciculation in any patient who might have motor neurone disease is always time well spent. Fasciculation in the tongue should be looked for with the tongue resting in the floor of the mouth. Fasciculation in calf muscles may be of no pathological significance.

In conclusion, the examination of any elderly patient is time-consuming and requires patience and great attention to detail. It may be necessary to go back to the patient on several occasions both to obtain a comprehensive history, and to be confident about abnormal neurological signs. Even after careful assessment it is sometimes not possible to come to definitive conclusions and it may be necessary to observe changes in physical signs over time. Serial observations, when properly recorded, are a cheaper method of reaching a diagnosis than scan or myelogram. For example, hemiparetic signs due to stroke tend to improve whereas those due to tumour progress. The evolution of the signs indicates the pathology. Likewise the rate of progression of paraparetic signs may help decide whether a patient with cervical spondylotic myelopathy can be managed conservatively in a collar or should be referred for assessment for neurosurgery.

2 The Investigation of the Elderly Patient

Progress in medicine makes for continuous changes in medical practice, but good clinical management, unlike politics, is not always the "art of the possible". Thus "high tech" medicine can achieve a definitive diagnosis in cases where previously there was only speculation or dogma. Treatment, including life support systems, pacemakers or transplant surgery, can prolong life in a way never before imagined. In neurology the diagnostic tools have advanced faster than the ability to restore neurological function and it is, therefore, often possible to achieve a definitive diagnosis, even if at substantial cost, without benefit to the patient. Clinicians have to be aware not only of what is possible in the way of investigatory techniques, but must also be informed of the prognosis in all situations. They must assess investigation and treatment against the background of increasing life expectancy and improving quality of life in the very elderly. It is important to have a knowledge of improvements in treatment, what can be achieved with modern anaesthesia and surgery in the old, and what support and rehabilitation facilities are available. It is not sufficient, therefore, to embark on complicated investigation to define a diagnosis without considering the individual patient in the longer perspective.

The elderly patient with neurological disability should have a "working diagnosis", because upon this depends the advice that can be given about prognosis and management. A "working diagnosis" need not commit the clinician; he should not feel that he has made a mistake if the diagnosis proves to be wrong. A working diagnosis provides a basis for action, but implies that alternative possibilities are borne in mind so that management policy and prognosis may be revised if necessary.

Failure to establish a "working diagnosis" from the outset leaves patient and relatives in a limbo of uncertainty and tempts the clinician to embark on unnecessary investigation. The patient and her family must expect assessment of the likely course of the disease process, what adjustments should be made to her environment and what treatment is available.

The decision, however, of when to use the definitive investigation is nearly always a very difficult one. At the two extremes the decision may be easy. Where it is a case of obvious malignant disease investigation may be not only wasteful but actually undermine the confidence of the relatives in the doctor's ability to manage the case. But where the patient is in good general health and there is high probability of a benign disorder, investigation, even in extreme old age, is often fully justified.

Case 2.1
A male of 73 years of age presented with weakness of his legs. On examination there was obvious widespread fasciculation, with wasting of the small hand muscles, brisk reflexes, extensor plantar responses and no sensory disturbance. Sphincter control was normal.

Although a diagnosis of motor neurone disease was accepted, investigation with a CT scan, myelography, and electromyography was ordered.

This should perhaps be contrasted with the following case.

Case 2.2
An 82-year-old female presented with progressive difficulty with walking, leading initially to frequent falls. She also had progressive impairment of bladder control. Over the twelve months after she was referred for out-patient assessment Mrs A.F. deteriorated, and required walking aids and ultimately admission to a nursing home when one leg became totally paralysed and she was wheelchair-bound.

Examination demonstrated paraplegia with a clear high thoracic sensory level, due to an extra-medullary tumour demonstrated on myelography.

Three weeks after surgery she was walking with two sticks and had regained sphincter control. And she was thereafter able to return to her own home and independent existence.

The appropriate investigation of the elderly patient can, therefore, only be planned on the basis of a careful examination and assessment of the patient and her environment and with a knowledge of a realistic treatment strategy.

It is unusual for some potentially treatable condition not to enter the differential diagnosis in most cases. General medicine, with its increasing reliance on definitive diagnostic investigation (and correspondingly diminishing trust in clinical skills) has taught many clinicians to order all investigations possibly relevant to the differential diagnosis. This strategy seldom applies in geriatric neurology because the definitive treatment (especially when surgical) may be inappropriate or frankly dangerous; and the investigation may cause discomfort and create possible hazard for the patient.

Relatives of the patient may insist on the need for "everything possible to be done" and as a result the doctor may very often feel disinclined to withold an investigation even though he is aware that it is unlikely to contribute useful information. It is very difficult to lead relatives in this situation to understand where the best interests of the patient lie, though it is important to try to do so. It must be accepted, however, that in institutions where non-invasive investigation such as scanning is readily available and where there is no direct cost to the patient, misuse of the service cannot always be avoided.

Any investigation that may lead to definitive treatment is mandatory unless it carries an unacceptably high risk to the patient. But where the result of the investigation is unlikely to lead to specific management decisions, two questions should be borne in mind:

1. Will the test allow an accurate prognosis to be given?
2. Will the results of the investigation have implications in terms of nursing care, therapy or rehabilitation?

The investigations that are commonly used in clinical neurology are lumbar puncture, CT scan, electroencephalography, electromyography and nerve conduction studies, evoked potential recording, myelography, angiography and MRI. The use of these investigations in the elderly patient will now be briefly reviewed.

Lumbar Puncture

This procedure is used to obtain information about the pressure and constituents of the cerebrospinal fluid (CSF), to introduce some contrast material for radiological investigation or to introduce therapeutic material, e.g., in leukaemic meningitis. The indications for the investigation of the CSF by lumbar puncture have changed since the introduction of CT scanning, both because lumbar puncture carries the risk of fatal "coning" if there is a space-occupying lesion within the cranium and because CT scanning can usually exclude a mass lesion, without risk.

In patients where the working diagnosis is subarachnoid haemorrhage or brain abscess (possibly associated with meningitis or vice versa) it is necessary to establish whether there is an intra-cerebral haematoma or abscess and whether there is displacement of the mid-line structures before lumbar puncture is carried out.

Lumbar puncture leads to a fall in the subarachnoid pressure in the lumbar region. Where a mass lesion is present the CSF pressure will be high. Posterior fossa masses may obstruct the foramen magnum and prevent equalisation of pressure in the spinal canal and head. The high pressure in the head drives the medulla and cerebellum into the foramen magnum and this may cause cardiac and respiratory arrest through "coning". Space-occupying lesions above the tentorium cerebelli, especially when lateralised, may cause a similar obstruction at the tentorial hiatus with posterior cerebral infarction, coma and death.

Thus there is an absolute contra-indication to lumbar puncture where there is the possibility of such a mass lesion. In the young, raised intracranial pressure usually gives rise to papilloedema which develops within 24–48 hours. But in the elderly this sign may be absent, even in the presence intracranially of a large lateralised mass; alternatively, the fundi may be obscured by cataract or other medial opacities. CT scanning is the essential preliminary to lumbar puncture in this situation.

There are two common acute problems where a knowledge of the CSF constituents is essential:

1. Where subarachnoid haemorrhage is suspected
2. Where meningitis is suspected

In either of these situations the CSF pressure may be raised. If CT scanning is readily available it should be done immediately and CSF obtained if the scan does not show any mass lesion. If no CT scan is immediately available (or if scanning will introduce delay) and there are no lateralising or posterior fossa neurological signs, then lumbar puncture should be carried out without delay. Failure to do so may make a critical difference to the outcome.

Subarachnoid haemorrhage (SAH) in the elderly most commonly, but by no means invariably, results from arteriosclerosis. Whereas surgical treatment of aneurysmal bleeds makes a substantial difference to the prognosis even in the elderly patient, arteriosclerotic or hypertensive subarachnoid haemorrhage is less likely to require surgical treatment and the management and prognosis are different. The distinction between these two types of subarachnoid bleeding has to be made on the basis of angiography (see below) but the diagnosis of subarachnoid bleeding can be made most easily and reliably by lumbar puncture.

The clinical diagnosis of subarachnoid haemorrhage can be very difficult.

Case 2.3
A 68-year-old female developed severe and increasing headache in the night after she had got out of bed to go to the toilet. Her symptoms were so severe that her husband summoned an ambulance and she was brought to Casualty. No abnormal signs could be found and she was sent home with analgesics. Because of severe persisting headache she was re-examined 12 hours later. There was still no detectable meningism but she was admitted and lumbar puncture revealed blood-stained CSF from an aneurysm which was later successfully clipped.

Note: It is usually wiser to admit and carry out a lumbar puncture procedure on a patient whose headache is due to benign causes than to send away a patient whose headache may be due to subarachnoid haemorrhage.

The outcome for a patient with meningitis is related closely to the delay between onset of the disease and starting treatment. Early diagnosis is, therefore, important and may be exceptionally difficult in the elderly where meningitis may present atypically (e.g., with confusion, hemiplegia or cortical blindness) and where signs, especially meningism, may be minimal or mimicked by conditions such as cervical spondylosis or dehydration. Lumbar puncture is the essential diagnostic procedure in meningitis and should always be done immediately, bearing in mind the contra-indications discussed already.

Chronic meningitis should be excluded by lumbar puncture in the elderly patient who presents with intractable undiagnosed headache of recent onset where there is no alternative explanation for the symptoms and especially where there are features consistent with the diagnosis. In old age, chronic meningitis tends to present with confusion, disturbance of balance and often with hemiplegia or ophthalmoplegia. Malignant meningitis is usually associated with very high protein and low sugar levels in the CSF. But the malignant cells may be difficult for the pathologist to identify unless his attention is specifically drawn to this possibility. It is essential to provide a fresh specimen and sufficient volume of CSF for a spun sample to be examined.

Measurement of CSF pressure is important in only a few situations in the elderly patient. In general, the pressure within the skull is affected later and less severely in the old, so that large mass lesions may be present without any rise of intracranial pressure. Benign intracranial hypertension is rare in old age. But "normal pressure hydrocephalus" enters the differential diagnosis in the patient with the triad of dementia, gait disturbance and incontinence. In such cases, where there is a past history of meningitis or subarachnoid haemorrhage and where CT scan has shown hydrocephalic changes, a knowledge of CSF pressure and constituents is necessary.

Computed Tomography (CT) Scan

The contra-indications to CT scan are almost solely related to considerations of economics and availability. Thus CT scanning is an expensive investigation and in most countries the availability of equipment is limited. The use of CT scan should, therefore, be limited to those cases where it is specifically indicated; that is, where there is clinical suspicion of a structural lesion intracranially, and the result will influence patient management.

For adequate visualisation of the intracranial structure the patient must keep still and there should be no metallic clips from previous neurosurgery. The patient has to be able to lie flat so that some patients with, for example, congestive cardiac failure may be unsuitable. In the case of a confused or restless patient who cannot lie still, general anaesthesia is necessary. In this case the gain from a CT scan has to be set against the risks of general anaesthesia as well as the added cost of a general anaesthetic. Considerations of this sort apply particularly in cases of dementia or subacute confusional states.

"Atrophic" changes on CT scan are the norm after 65 years of age. Thus, in the geriatric age groups widening of the subarachnoid space and sulci is evident and some degree of enlargement of the ventricles is the rule. These changes correlate poorly with brain function so that advanced atrophic changes may be found in someone who shows normal higher mental function; and similarly CT atrophy may be absent or slight in a case of advanced dementia. The value of a scan in the dementing patient is to exclude mass lesions or disturbance of CSF hydrodynamics as the cause for the dementia.

Head injury is a common indication for CT scan, either where an immediate assessment of brain injury is required in the patient who has been concussed, or where there is a likelihood of chronic subdural haematoma. Any patient suspected of cerebral tumour who is not known to have a malignant primary outside the head should be scanned if her condition allows. Only in this way can the diagnosis be safely confirmed, a prognosis given, and a plan made for the management of the condition.

The subsequent neurosurgical management may require further CT or other investigation.

There is much discussion and argument about the use of CT scanning in patients with headache or those who have suffered their first epileptic fit. Where scanning facilities are readily available, a patient with recent onset headache without obvious or certain cause should probably be scanned. Headache is discussed in more detail elsewhere but it is rare for headache to be due to structural intracranial cause without there being any suspicious feature in the history or on examination. It is important to realise that a normal CT scan does not exclude a structural cause for the headache. Bilateral subdural haematoma, aneurysm and basal meningiomas may be "missed" on the scan and lead to false complacency. It is more important, therefore, to assess the patient carefully by a detailed history and physical examination than to press for a CT scan.

Epilepsy "of late onset" is also discussed elsewhere in this volume, but in general the scan is less helpful than the EEG in demonstrating abnormality, unless there are clinical features indicative of a focal cerebral abnormality. Where this is so, a CT scan is indicated.

The patient presenting with signs of hemiparesis may pose the common problem: is it a tumour or is it a stroke? It is seldom appropriate to scan such cases. The diagnosis is made by the evolution of the signs – strokes get better, tumours do not. And the delay in diagnosis of a tumour presenting as stroke seldom alters the management. It is noteworthy that dexamethasone usually produces a more impressive temporary improvement in symptoms in patients with cerebral tumour than it does in those recovering from stroke.

Although CT scan will seldom provide a definitive explanation it should be done in cases of undiagnosed coma because unexpected pathology in brainstem, temporal lobes or elsewhere may thereby be revealed. A normal scan never provides any reassurance since most of the causes of coma are disturbances of brain function (toxic, metabolic or electrical) that do not give rise to any abnormality of structure of the brain.

Electroencephalography (EEG)

As with CT scanning, EEG is a non-invasive procedure so that the constraints on its use are those of economics and availability. They are also the perception of the clinician of the value of this investigation, and this is where misunderstanding may arise. The EEG provides a relatively poor guide to brain structure, poor, that is, in comparison to CT scanning. What the EEG does provide is a demonstration of the electrical function of the brain at the time the record was taken. It follows that any ongoing disturbance of electrical function will be best demonstrated by EEG: coma, for instance, as has been noted above.

Epilepsy may give rise to no continuing electrical disturbance of the brain (40% of EEGs in patients with definite epilepsy show no paroxysmal disturbance). The attacks may be separated by entirely normal brain function, not only clinically but also on EEG. Thus EEG is not always helpful in the diagnosis of epilepsy or, to put it differently, a normal EEG does not disclose whether the "attack" was epileptic or not. The diagnosis must be made on clinical grounds. But an EEG taken in a patient who has had one or more epileptic seizures may show an abnormality indicating the type of epilepsy. Thus the EEG may be generally abnormal or it may have a single focus of abnormality or many separate foci. If the abnormality is generalised the pattern may have diagnostic features, for example, those of primary generalised epilepsy or those of a degenerative encephalopathy. A focal EEG abnormality may provide the indication of focal pathology required to justify a CT scan, in a patient with late onset epilepsy. Multi-focal abnormalities are consistent with, and therefore supportive of, a diagnosis of multi-infarct brain disease, multiple metastases or vasculitis.

The EEG records the electrical potentials from the surface of the cerebral hemispheres – the cortex of the gyri. It does not pick up abnormalities of the cortex in the sulci and still less abnormalities in the deeper structures of the brain. Disturbances of the white matter, or brainstem, may be reflected in projected abnormalities of EEG which cause changes in the cortical potentials, but these projected abnormalities tend to be non-specific slowing of normal rhythms.

In the investigation of the elderly patient EEG may fail to show diagnostic abnormality even where otherwise the features of the disease are typical. For example, a patient with Jakob–Creutzfeldt disease may never show the repetitive complexes described in the textbook. A "negative" EEG should seldom be taken as evidence against a diagnosis whereas the opposite – that is, positive

Table 2.1. Cardinal indications for EEG in the elderly

1. *Epilepsy*
     ? Focal: e.g., brain tumour, infarct etc.
     ? Multi-focal: e.g., multi-infarct, vasculopathy, multiple metastases
     ? Specific: e.g., primary generalised epilepsy, Jakob–Creutzfeldt disease
     Note: If an attack occurs spontaneously or can be induced during the recording, then:
     a. The diagnosis of epilepsy can be confirmed
     b. Information about the type of epilepsy can be obtained
     c. A precipitating cause may be identifiable: e.g., photic stimulation, hypoglycaemia.
2. *Coma or Stupor*
     ? Generalised: e.g., encephalopathy
     ? Generalised but assymmetrical or focal: e.g., encephalitis
     ? Minor epileptic status
3. *Dementia*
     ? non specific, low voltage with excess slow: e.g., Alzheimer's disease or Huntington's chorea
     ? Specific: e.g., Jakob–Creutzfeldt disease
     ? focal: e.g., frontal tumour
4. *Other*
     e.g., sleep apnoea, hepatic failure, other metabolic disorders

and typical abnormalities – can be taken as strong evidence in support of a diagnosis.

The cardinal indications for EEG in the elderly are summarised in the Table 2.1.

EEG recording cannot be carried out satisfactorily if the patient is restless or unco-operative. It is important to advise the EEG Department if the patient has had a recent fit or is taking sedative medication; it is not necessary to stop anticonvulsant drugs before an EEG trace is recorded.

The EEG is normally reported with an opinion offered by the clinical neurophysiologist. This opinion will always be more reliable if all the clinical information for requesting an EEG is given on the request form.

Electromyography (EMG) and Nerve Conduction Velocity (NCV)

Few clinicians have detailed knowledge or experience of these techniques and are, therefore, uncertain of their indications. This is unfortunate since EMG and NCV can provide information about muscle and peripheral nerve function which is most valuable in assessment, diagnosis and treatment.

Electromyography is the recording of resting activity and muscle action potentials, usually through a needle electrode in the muscle. It is, therefore, restricted to those muscles that are accessible, so that the diaphragm, constrictor muscles of the pharynx or the pelvic muscles are seldom investigated. From the potentials recorded from the muscle at rest and on voluntary contraction it is usually possible to identify:

1. Denervation,
2. Myopathy,
3. Fasciculation potentials in motor neurone disease,
4. Myotonia

EMG may, therefore, allow the crucial distinction to be made about the cause of the weakness: is it due to nerve damage, and to muscle disease or is it apparent weakness secondary to pain from a joint? Where fasciculation potentials can be demonstrated by EMG but are not evident clinically, and where these abnormal potentials are present at several widely separated segmental levels a diagnosis of motor neurone disease is almost certain.

The EMG features indicating myopathy may provide an indication for muscle biopsy leading to a definitive diagnosis. Whereas myasthenia gravis may be easier to diagnose clinically than by EMG, myasthenic syndrome (Eaton–Lambert syndrome) can only be confirmed by these methods.

Nerve conduction studies are indicated for the diagnosis of peripheral poly- or mono-neuropathies. NCV is useful on three counts

1. It provides measure of the rate of nerve conduction so that the severity of the disorder and its evolution in time can be determined
2. It gives information about the localisation of a focal lesion on a peripheral nerve. Or when the lesion is proximal (i.e., at the nerve root) it gives an indication of whether it is proximal or distal to the dorsal root ganglion. (Note that cervical spondylotic root lesions are proximal to the dorsal root ganglion. Most other causes of radiculopathy are distal.)
3. It indicates whether the neuropathy is generalised, that is, is likely to be primarily:
   a. axonal (and therefore due to toxic or nutritional causes; or motor neurone disease in the case of a pure motor neuropathy)
   b. demyelinating, e.g., Guillain–Barré syndrome
   c. associated with fibrosis of the perineurium as in leprosy

Thus NCV is a useful lead to definitive diagnosis in disorders of peripheral nerve. But it is not necessary to have nerve conduction studies where the diagnosis can be made on clinical grounds. Carpal tunnel syndrome or ulnar neuropathy at the elbow can usually be diagnosed without recourse to NCV.

Evoked Potential Recording

The primary use of evoked potential recording is in the diagnosis of multiple sclerosis. This condition seldom presents in the elderly. But occasionally patients will present with paraparesis of uncertain aetiology, where the possibility of multiple sclerosis exists and where visual or brainstem evoked potentials may give the clue to other lesions disseminated in the central nervous system.

Myelography

It is likely that myelography will increasingly be superceded by MRI scanning (see below) but until this form of scanning is widely available myelography remains the essential investigation of any patient suspected of having a structural compressive lesion of the spinal cord or cauda equina. In geriatric practice, weakness of the legs, difficulty with walking and mild signs of pyramidal deficit are commonplace. The association of bladder disturbance with reduced or absent lower limb reflexes may suggest the possibility of a cauda equina lesion.

Most elderly patients will admit to backache or pain in the neck even if they do not volunteer this symptom. And finally the sensory examination of the very old requires patience and perseverance. A clinical diagnosis of spinal or cauda equina lesion is the first essential preliminary to myelography. The second preliminary is the question "if we find a compressive lesion will the patient tolerate and benefit from its removal?" Thus myelography carries the presupposition that it is a preliminary to neurosurgery if the investigation is positive.

Myelography is unpleasant for the patient whose co-operation has to be maintained for more than half an hour. She has to tolerate a lumbar puncture under local anaesthetic, a tilt table and usually subsequent CT scanning of the spine. But in addition to providing a detailed radiological image of the spinal canal and its contents, myelography provides a specimen of CSF for analysis thereby adding an extra dimension to the information derived.

Any compressive lesion found on myelography may cause acute deterioration following myelography. If the neurosurgeon has not been told of the case before myelography he should be informed immediately a compressive lesion is found so that the patient can be prepared for surgery with the appropriate urgency.

Elderly patients tolerate spinal surgery remarkably well so that myelography or a surgical opinion should be sought even in the very old disabled patient where spinal compression is suspected. The alternative is the prolonged nursing care of a paraplegic. However, acute spinal lesions in the aged are commonly due to extradural metastases and therefore it is important to investigate a patient with acute cord compression urgently for a primary neoplasm and thereby save them the need for myelography. Decompression of extradural metastases is seldom justified unless to relieve pain. Where no primary malignancy is found, urgent myelography is necessary to make the diagnosis and exclude some acute treatable lesion such as prolapsed disc. An important part of the examination of the acute elderly paraplegic is an assessment of the arteries to the lower limbs – pulses and bruits and palpation for abdominal aortic aneurysm. Dissection of the aorta with occlusion of the lumbar arteries supplying the spinal cord is an important cause of acute paraplegia and diagnosis may save the patient a myelogram.

Angiography

Even where modern apparatus for digital subtraction techniques is available, angiography usually requires a general anaesthetic. As with myelography, therefore, angiography should normally be considered a preliminary to neurovascular surgery but, unlike spinal surgery, intracranial neurovascular surgery is poorly tolerated by the old. The decision to investigate an elderly patient with an intracranial haemorrhage, an aneurysm or arterio-venous fistula must be a neurosurgical decision. The responsibility of the physician is to make the working diagnosis and this is dealt with elsewhere in this book.

Angiography is sometimes queried for the investigation of the patient presenting with transient ischaemic attacks or even completed stroke who has a bruit in the neck or reduced blood pressure in one arm (suggesting the possibility of a subclavian steal syndrome). Again it must be emphasised that investigation of such a patient presupposes that she will tolerate and benefit from disobliterative surgery. The epidemiological data to demonstrate the benefits of surgery in such cases are at present lacking. Medical treatment without recourse to angiography is usually the appropriate management at this age.

Similar considerations apply in cases of intracerebral or subarachnoid haemorrhage; or where aneurysm presents with the classical features of posterior communicating artery aneurysm (lateralised frontal pain, partial IIIrd nerve palsy, and sensory loss in ophthalmic V). The operative mortality from aneurysm surgery in patients over 60 years old approaches 50%.

The procedure of angiography carries a significant morbidity with risk of transient hemiparetic symptoms or other evidence of disturbed cerebral perfusion occurring in 2%–5% of elderly cases. This risk is greatly increased where there is spasm of blood vessels or in the presence of hypertension.

Magnetic Resonance Imaging (MRI)

This technique is non-invasive and allows better imaging than CT at bone/soft tissue interfaces. It also allows imaging in the sagittal and coronal planes. MRI may be expected gradually to displace CT for the investigation of the orbit, midline and especially basal intracranial lesions, and the spinal canal at all levels. As with all forms of imaging done with the patient conscious, co-operation and the ability to keep still is necessary. The image is not distorted by metallic clips (as it is with CT) but attention has to be paid to the possibility of damage from metallic clips within the skull moving as the result of the high magnetic field. Otherwise there is no known hazard. However, MRI is expensive and is likely to remain so. Selection criteria for this investigation must, therefore, remain rigorous. These criteria are the same as those discussed for CT scanning.

3 "Confusion" and Dementia

The term "confusion" is used loosely to describe any recent disturbance of higher mental function. Strictly speaking "confusion" means "lack of clarity of thought" – which may better describe the mind of the doctor than that of his patient. It is usually preferable to describe the patient as having an "impaired mental state", which must then be defined in terms of her cognitive, affective and behavioural abnormalities.

There is some difficulty in defining the "normal" in elderly patients, many of whom admit to difficulty in remembering recent information in contrast to excellent recall of specific events 20 or more years previously. Absent-mindedness exemplified by going upstairs to fetch something and then forgetting what she has gone to fetch, is very common, but is also found amongst much younger individuals. The extent to which this is a "lack of use" phenomenon as opposed to true cognitive decline may be very unclear when the impairment is mild, but patients and relatives may seek urgent medical reassurance about such symptoms because they fear the onset of a dementing process. Many patients presenting in this way show no evidence of cognitive impairment on formal testing.

The true situation may only become apparent over the course of time, progressive impairment indicating an underlying organic process. A careful clinical approach with, if necessary, follow-up assessment after an interval will generally resolve the diagnostic dilemma.

Many elderly patients exhibit impairment in mental function at the time of presentation to medical services. These may be a direct reflection of an acute underlying illness – an acute organic brain syndrome (sometimes referred to as delirium, a toxic confusional state, or acute organic psychosyndrome). Though a patient with an acute organic brain syndrome may superficially resemble someone who is demented, the implications are very different. The former may be due to severe life-threatening physical illness, and the impairment would then be expected to clear with recovery, whereas in dementia the impairment in mental function will have been progressive over time. In confusional states, diagnosis and treatment is directed towards acute cerebral or general disease. In dementia the definitive diagnosis is made to exclude treatable causes and to give a prognosis on which management may be planned.

Thus the recent onset of impaired mental state in elderly patients will usually indicate that special investigation should be undertaken to answer the following questions. Has a previously mildly impaired individual who suddenly appears very demented developed some general systemic disorder such as an infection or cardiac failure? Has a gradual dementing process been overlooked until some critical abnormal behaviour (e.g., incontinence) brought it to notice? Are there features to suggest a specific or focal disorder of brain function (e.g., stroke, Huntington's chorea, or a frontal space-occupying lesion)?

In Chapter 2 emphasis is placed on the need for co-operation by the patient (and often her family) if special investigations such as scanning or EEG are to be done. Similarly, successful physiotherapy and mobilisation depends on a degree of co-operation by the patient and also on the patient being able to remember from moment to moment and from day to day what the therapist has told her.

History

A systematic approach is important in the proper management of impaired mental function in the elderly. The history should always be obtained from someone who has close knowledge of the patient. A past history of psychiatric disorder, mental subnormality, epilepsy or alcohol excess is important and a history of the patient's medication is essential. The patient herself need only be asked about specific mental or physical symptoms. It is usually more acceptable to the patient for the doctor to first enquire of her regarding physical symptoms (headaches, dizziness, sleep) and then ask about mental symptoms (hallucinations, depression, memory and ideas of reference). Where the relative or friend indicates that there has been behaviour suggestive of dementia or a confusional state, specific examples should always be sought. Where and under what emotional stress did the patient get lost or forgetful? What precise behaviour was considered abnormal? What skill is the patient now no longer actually capable of? What abnormal activity or emotional state do they now exhibit? Finally the patient's previous occupation, hobbies and interests may indicate significant deterioration from a previously highly intelligent level.

Case 3.1
A highly intelligent retired schoolteacher was found to have a measured IQ of 110 at the time of presentation. But a personality change with obstreporous argumentative behaviour coupled with a mild memory disturbance heralded the onset of a dementia of the Alzheimer type.

Prior to examining the patient, getting her into as relaxed and comfortable a state as possible is essential. Many "confused" old people are best interviewed in the familiar surroundings of their own home, though this may not always be possible. The patient should be seated so as to be able to see the face of the doctor and should be wearing spectacles and hearing aid if necessary. If she wishes to empty her bladder or bowel she should be toileted before the start of the interview. The doctor should introduce himself and tell her why he is seeing her and the interview should not be rushed. It may be necessary to conduct several shorter interviews in order that the patient does not become over-tired and even more muddled. Occasionally observation in hospital may be necessary and more valuable than several out-patient attendances. An informal approach to the patient and chatting about her life, where she lives and her children, not only gives the patient confidence but may elicit valuable information and may help to gain an overall impression of what the mental state is. Special note can be taken at this stage of dysphasic symptoms, memory defect, affective disturbance and abnormal involuntary movements such as myoclonus, tremor or chorea. Confabulation is usually indicative of pathology affecting the mammillary bodies especially Wernicke's encephalopathy.

The mode of onset often provides the clue to causation. If the history is short the patient is suffering from an acute confusional state usually due to a physical illness, for example an acute infection, heart failure or an injury. Primary brain disorder may be the cause of the acute confusional state but in general the process is likely to be diffuse or multifocal rather than a focal brain disorder such as stroke.

Meningitis, encephalitis and subarachnoid haemorrhage may present in the elderly as an acute confusional state and may require early lumbar puncture for diagnosis. Pituitary lesions may present especially in the old as a progressing confusional state with apathy, vagueness and memory failure.

She may have a "pseudodementia" – a presentation of depression or other functional psychiatric illnesses in the elderly described later in the chapter. A recent bereavement (including the loss of pets) or change in lifestyle (for example, a move to institutional care) may have been important in precipitating a depressive illness with agitated restless and confused behaviour.

The clinical features of the mental state may provide diagnostic information, but it is important to remember that relatives and neighbours sometimes misinterpret what is happening. For example, they may describe the patient as being "very forgetful" when in reality the patient has dysphasia or is dressing incorrectly due to dyspraxia. Does the patient truly have impairment of memory or disorientation in time, place or person? Has the patient been deluded; if so, is this accompanied by memory loss or disorientation (in which case an acute organic brain syndrome or underlying dementia are likely) or are the delusions occurring in isolation (in which case a functional psychiatric disorder is more likely)? Visual hallucinations are more suggestive of acute organic syndromes (or related to drug therapy) whereas auditory hallucinations tend to be associated with psychotic conditions. In acute confusional states, whether due to systemic disorder or primary brain syndromes, there is usually some reduction of alertness or impairment of consciousness. In psychotic conditions the thought disorder is in a clear alert sensorium.

Drugs are a potent cause of impaired mental state in the elderly and will be discussed in some detail later. The importance of an accurate, recent, drug

Table 3.1. Important points in the history in an elderly patient with altered mental function

1. *Mode of onset:*
   When did the patient's mental state change?
   Was the onset sudden or gradual?
2. *The progress of the condition over time:*
   Has the patient's mental state stayed the same, become worse, improved or fluctuated?
3. *Clinical features of the mental state*
   Memory
   Disorientation
   Delusions
   Hallucinations
4. *Past and family history and patient's previous medical and psychiatric illnesses:*
   Has the patient had a similar problem in the past? If so, when and how often?
   Family illnesses
5. *Current drug history*
   Has the patient been taking any medication recently? (It may be necessary to ask for the medicaments to be brought in to the hospital, or to contact the general practitioner for further details.)
   How much alcohol does the patient consume?
6. *The patient's previous mental capacity*
   What is the patient's memory normally like and how was it in years past? (Important in determining the presence of low intelligence.)

history cannot be over-emphasised. It is urgent and the general practitioner should, if necessary, be contacted by telephone.

Specific enquiry should be made for a history of fits or other transient neurological symptoms. Thus a history of dysphasia or paresis or sensory loss in the face or limbs may be indicative of a focal brain disturbance. The important points in the history of an elderly patient with altered mental function are given in Table 3.1.

Examination

In the course of history-taking cognitive impairment may be evident. The content of speech and language during spontaneous conversation may provide clues to the presence of dysphasia, functional psychiatric illness and delusional and hallucinatory states, and sometimes to abnormalities of praxis and attention.

There is always a dilemma in assessing cognition in patients who may be only mildly impaired. The patient may resent being asked what may seem rather absurdly easy or pointless questions and it is important to introduce formal testing of memory function with appropriate words such as "I'm going to ask you a few questions which may perhaps seem to you to be a bit silly but which are nevertheless important in making sure that you are remembering things clearly".

The examination of a patient's mental state should be structured so that the organic is distinguished from the psychiatric; and the focal from the generalised disturbance of brain function. Behaviour (including general appearance, tidiness and hygiene) content of thought (delusions, hallucinations, ideas of reference) and mood (depressed, agitated or elated) should each be separately noted. These are the cardinal signs of psychiatric disorder but may be present in organic brain syndromes when they tend to be associated with an abnormality of cognitive function (see Table 3.2).

Cognitive function should be assessed first by recording the patient's orientation in time (day, date, month, season, year) and place (present whereabouts and home address). Conscious awareness and attention should next be considered. Drowsiness is easily detected but minor degrees of distractability or somnolence may be more difficult to detect (see Chap. 9). These signs are the general indications of diffuse organic disturbance of brain function. Focal disturbance will cause abnormalities of cognitive function including (either alone or in combination) memory impairment, language disorder (dysphasia, dyslexia, dysgraphia) visuo-spatial disability and constructional dyspraxia.

Tests of Memory

A few simple tests should establish whether there is a severe defect of memory or of immediate recall. The name address and flower test gives 7 items of which the patient should be able to repeat 4 or 5 after 5 minutes: "Michael (1) Robinson (2) 37 (3) West (4) Drive (5) Swindon (6) Primrose (7)".

The Babcock sentence should be correctly repeated after three or four repetitions: "One thing a nation must have to be rich and great is a large secure supply of wood".

Table 3.2. Diagnostic pointers in elderly patients with impaired mental state

Cognitive Impairment plus:
1. Disorientation, drowsiness and inattention
   Acute or subacute Organic Brain Syndrome
   or
2. Memory impairment, dysphasia or visuo-spatial disorientation
   Alzheimer's disease or Focal brain disease
   or
3. Thought disorder, abnormal mood, appearance and behaviour
   Psychiatric, Nutritional or toxic states
   or
4. Akinetic-rigid state, supranuclear opthalmoplegia, chorea, strokes or amyotrophy
   Specific dementias.

Table 3.3. The Abbreviated Mental Test (Qureshi and Hodkinson 1974). Each correct answer scores one mark)

1. Patient's age
2. Time (correct to nearest hour)
3. Address for recall at end of the test – it should be repeated by the patient to ensure it has been heard correctly: "42 West Street"
4. Year
5. Name of hospital (or place of current residence)
6. Recognition of two persons (doctor, nurse etc)
7. Date of birth
8. Year of the First World War
9. Name of present monarch
10. Count backwards 20–1

A score of 7 or less suggests cognitive impairment.

Memory of current affairs and general information (dates of World War II, names of Queen's children etc.) can be easily tested and assessed for significant impairment.

One of the most widely used measures of cognitive function is the Abbreviated Mental Test (AMT) of Qureshi and Hodkinson (1974). The test is easy to apply and has been found to be very reliable. The questions are listed in Table 3.3.

Tests of Language Function

Spontaneous speech should be carefully assessed for vocabulary, syntax, speed or hesitation and mispronunciations or neologisms. Specific naming tests of common objects should be graduated with increasing difficulty if mild dysphasia is suspected ("watch" "face" "winder" "buckle"; or "spectacles", "lens", "bridge", "hinge"). Similarly, receptive dysphasia should be tested first with simple tests – "close your eyes", "hold out your hands" and then graduated to more difficult tests "tear this paper into three. Give me one piece, put another in your pocket and throw the third on the floor".

Writing can be tested first to dictation and then by asking the patient to describe the weather or what she likes for breakfast; and finally reading can be tested by asking the patient to read a simple instruction and testing for comprehension. The Mini-Mental State examination (Table 3.4) provides a simple and useful score of cognitive function.

Visuo-spatial Disorientation

Ask the patient to copy simple diagrams, such as Fig. 3.1, or to draw a bicycle or clock face. Note especially if she tends to ignore the left half of the diagram and crowds detail to the right, which may suggest a right parietal lesion.

 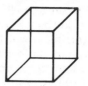

Fig. 3.1

Table 3.4. The "mini-mental state" (Folstein et al. 1975)

Maximum Score	Score	
		Orientation
5	( )	What is the (year) (season) (date) (month)?
5	( )	Where are we: (country) (county) (town) (hospital) (ward)?
		Registration
3	( )	Name 3 objects: 1 second to say each. Then ask the patient all 3 after you have said them. Give 1 point for each correct answer. Then repeat them until he learns all 3. Count trials and record. Trials. . . . .
		Attention and calculation
5	( )	Serial 7s (subtract 7 from 100 and keep doing it). 1 point for each correct. Stop after 5 answers. Alternatively spell "world" backwards
		Recall
3	( )	As for the 3 objects repeated above. Give 1 point for each correct
		Language and copying
9	( )	Name a pencil, and a watch (2 points)
	( )	Repeat the following: "No ifs, ands, or buts" (1 point)
	( )	Follow a 3-stage command: "Pick up a paper with your right hand, fold it in half, and put it on the floor" (3 points)
	( )	Read and obey the following: "Close your eyes" (1 point)
		Write a sentence (1 Point) Copy a design (1 point)
30		Total score
		Assess level of consciousness along a continuum
		Alert Drowsy Stupor Coma

A score of less than 20 is highly suggestive of cognitive impairment: demented patients tend to score below 10.

Physical Examination

Any elderly patient presenting with impaired mental function requires a full physical examination. Physical illness may be the cause of the behavioural change or, in patients with pre-existing psychiatric disorder, may aggravate the mental state. Thus a patient with a respiratory tract infection may develop an acute brain syndrome and may become behaviourally disturbed for the first time; or the infection may, through the superimposition of an acute brain syndrome in an already demented patient, lead to wandering, aggression or nocturnal disturbance. The presence of physical illness may also fundamentally affect the treatment which the patient has for her mental illness. Thus a patient with depression and coexisting ischaemic heart disease may respond adversely to tricyclic antidepressants and alternative medication should be considered. The issue of physical fitness for electroconvulsive therapy may also arise.

Acute and Subacute Organic Brain Syndromes

Delirium is extremely common in the hospitalised elderly and is associated with a high mortality. In studies of patients over the age of 65 years admitted to geriatric wards the incidence of acute confusional states at the time of admission has ranged between 35% and 80%; this wide range probably reflects different patterns of working in the units involved in these studies. In elderly patients admitted to general medical wards the incidence is of the order of 16%. About 25% of elderly patients thought to be cognitively intact at admission develop delirium during the first month of hospitalisation. Between 10% and 15% of elderly patients undergoing general surgery suffer post-operative acute confusion, and in patients admitted with fracture of the femoral neck, acute confusion at admission or during the subsequent period of hospitalisation affects about 60%. The mortality of patients with delirium during the index admission has been found to be between 25% and 33%. Many of the clinical features have already been described. Common causes of these conditions are listed in Table 3.5.

Acute organic brain syndromes are characterised by the sudden onset of cognitive impairment, disorientation, fluctuating impaired awareness, disruption of the sleep–wake cycle and, in severe cases, delusions and hallucinations. There is always underlying physical disease or drug intoxication though this may be little evident. The search for the underlying cause, if not obvious, is urgent in view of the high mortality found in this condition. Treatment should begin immediately and should include not only the underlying disorder but also secondary physical changes (for example dehydration arising in a patient with a chest infection). If treatment is effective it will hopefully be accompanied by improvement of the mental state over a few days but often in elderly people recovery is slow. During recovery the patient may pass through a phase when, despite continuing impairment, she begins to have increasing insight into (and memory of) her mental disturbance; this can be taken as a sign of improvement. Failure to improve should always lead to full reassessment of the patient's condition and the effectiveness of the management.

Pituitary apoplexy, where there is a haemorrhagic infarction of a pituitary tumour may present as an acute confusional state in a patient who will usually show some physical signs of endocrine disturbance (hypopituitarism or acromegaly). Pituitary apoplexy is associated with collapse and shock and, on neurological examination, ophthalmoplegia. This neurological sign may be

Table 3.5. The causes of acute and chronic organic brain syndromes in the elderly.

	Acute confusion	Dementia
Degenerative	Dementia complicated by infection, cardiac, respiratory disorder etc.	Alzheimer's; Diffuse Lewy Body disease (senile parkinsonism) Creutzfeldt–Jakob, Huntington's chorea; progressive supra-nuclear palsy, progressive multi-focal leucoencephalopathy, dementia of frontal type (with or without amyotrophy)
Vascular	Stroke, transient ischaemic attack, subarachnoid haemorrhage, hypertensive encephalopathy	Multi-infarct dementia; subcortical arterio-sclerotic encephalopathy (Binswanger's disease)
Metabolic	Hepatic failure, electrolyte disturbance, remote effects of carcinoma, uraemia, hypoglycaemia	Liver disorder
Toxic	Alcohol-Wernicke's encephalopathy, delerium tremens, barbiturates or benzodiazepines etc. anaesthetics	Alcoholic dementia, chronic sedative intoxication
Anoxic	Pneumonia, Cardiac failure, dysrrhythmia or infarction, occult haemorrhage, (e.g., gastrointestinal tract)	Anaemia, post cardiac arrest, CO poisoning
Nutritional	Wernicke's encephalopathy	Thiamine deficiency, pellagra, B_{12}, folate deficiency, cachexia
Others	Space-occupying lesion, encephalitis or meningitis, septicaemia, post ictal, endocrine esp. Addisonian crisis or acute hypo-pituitarism	Space-occupying lesion Chronic subdural haematoma, chronic encephalitis, hypothyroidism, G.P.I. normal pressure hydrocephalus pseudodementia

easily overlooked in the restless, confused patient. Radiography of the skull will often reveal enlargement of the pituitary fossa.

In subacute states the general picture is similar to that of acute states except that the onset of the condition is more insidious, its severity less than that found in the acute states (in which the behavioural changes are often florid) and the underlying physical cause less obvious. The fluctuation may occur over a longer period of time, the patient sometimes having "good times" in each day or even "good days and bad days".

Case 3.2

A 69-year-old female was known to have suffered from Parkinson's disease for 3 years, which responded poorly to a number of anti-parkinsonian drugs. The patient was admitted for assessment and rehabilitation. Several days after commencing a small dose (1'mg nocte) of bromocriptine she became muddled and exhibited marked paranoid ideation. This was initially thought to be due to bromocriptine, which was therefore withdrawn. The behavioural change persisted and further physical assessment revealed a variable blood pressure and repeat chest X-ray examinations showed cardiomegaly with upper lobe blood diversion.

At this time the patient had no other physical evidence of left ventricular failure. Treatment with frusemide was accompanied by a rapid improvement in the patient's mental and physical state. At this stage she tolerated bromocriptine without any recurrence of the impaired mental state.

Little is known of the mechanisms underlying acute and subacute organic brain syndromes. Disturbances in salt, water and calcium metabolism have been implicated. It is probably the "final common pathway" of expression of a variety of disruptions of brain function, including those associated with alterations in cerebral arousal, metabolism, blood flow and oxygenation, together with, in stroke or other focal disease, areas of damaged brain tissue. Some authorities believe that such a reaction to underlying physical illness (or to medication) represents the effect of the condition on a brain that is already subclinically damaged and which is, therefore, more susceptible to a variety of metabolic derangements and to drug therapy than the normal brain.

Investigation of any of these states must include a full blood count, an ESR or C-reactive protein, serum urea and electrolytes, blood sugar, serum calcium, tests of thyroid and hepatic function, a chest X-ray examination and a mid-stream specimen of urine for microscopy and culture. Each abnormality should be pursued since the acute mental change may reflect several abnormalities rather than one and all should, if possible, be corrected. Where there is suspicion of intracranial cause, EEG, lumbar puncture, skull X-ray and CT scan may be necessary.

Confusional States due to Drugs

Drug handling by the body and tissue responsiveness change with increasing age and poor compliance with treatment (either too little or too much medication) compound the problem. Drug interactions are more common in the elderly as is polypharmacy. The range of drugs used in the elderly include those with potent physical and behavioural side effects. Hypotensive, anti-parkinsonian drugs for dizziness and psychotropic agents carry considerable risks. Anticholinergic agents are particularly prone to cause confusion in the elderly; this probably arises as a result of their effect on the cholinergic pathways involved in cognition which are specifically affected in dementia of the Alzheimer type.

Nocturnal Behavioural Disturbance

This can occur in many situations and can be particularly troublesome in patients with dementia. In some patients, however, there may be a striking contrast between the normality of the mental state during the day and the presence of disturbed behaviour at night. Most such patients have a subacute organic brain syndrome. This may be due to drugs (including hypnotics and antidepressants), nocturnal left ventricular failure presenting with acute brain syndrome (rather than with the more common breathlessness or nocturnal angina), nocturnal hypoglycaemia (usually due to hypoglycaemic agents and much more rarely to insulinoma) or to nocturnal epilepsy. Description of the attack by nursing staff is not enough to establish the diagnosis; medical examination of the patient during such an episode is essential if treatable causes are not to be missed. Investigations include chest X-ray examination during the day (since most patients with nocturnal left ventricular failure will have radiological changes in the daytime), blood sugar during the episode, and EEG, if necessary by ambulatory monitoring techniques.

Nutritional and Toxic Confusional States

Disorders of memory are considered later (See Chap. 9). But a number of defined syndromes cause acute or subacute disorders of mental function and may present as a confusional state with the memory defect not immediately clinically obvious. Nutritional deficiency, often associated with the toxic effect of alcohol, is the usual cause of these syndromes. They are frequently seen in the elderly where early senile changes, poverty and social isolation lead to impairment of self care.

Pellagra or nicotinic acid deficiency may develop slowly with the early features easily dismissed as senile changes. Lethargy – both mental and physical – is characteristic and is usually associated with equally non-specific symptoms such as depression, irritability and emotional instability. In the elderly, ample financial resources may be no bar to the consumption of a grossly inadequate diet (and the affluent are commonly more prone to chronic alcoholic excess).

Pellagra is easily memorised as the triad of "diarrhoea, dementia and dermatitis" but this alliteration overlooks the important diagnostic features which are:

1. The diarrhoea is typically associated with glossitis and stomatitis
2. The dementia is characteristically associated with a short-term memory defect (unlike Alzheimer's disease where the memory defect also involves remote memory)
3. The "dermatitis" is a pigmentation of the skin especially involving bony prominences with reddening of the dorsum of the hands

Central pontine myelinolysis is a rare cause of acute confusional state associated with tetraplegia and often with pseudobulbar palsy. The demyelination of the pyramidal tracts in the pons seems to result from too rapid correction of a low sodium state complicating severe vomiting, alcoholism, or inappropriate antidiuretic hormone secretion. Although hitherto this condition has carried a very bad prognosis, remyelination of the pyramidal tracts with recovery of the spastic tetraplegia and recovery of the mental changes will take place if the patient is saved from intercurrent complications.

The chronic toxic effects of alcohol on the nervous system are considered in more detail in Chapter 11. They cause an acute confusional state (delirium tremens) and a dementia (alcoholic cerebral atrophy). Delirium tremens is seen less often in the elderly than in the middle-aged or younger patient. But alcoholic dementia is not uncommon in the old, where it is often complicated by the nutritional deficiencies already discussed. In some cases a lifetime of relatively high consumption of alcohol appears quite abruptly to give way to intolerance of the drug and a progressive decline in mental function. The features of the dementia tend to be "frontal" but with associated memory impairment. Thus there is disinhibited behaviour and social disintegration, often with preservation of a reasonable facade covering a severe memory defect. Abstinence, surprisingly, may lead to substantial recovery but unfortunately is seldom achieved.

Marchiafava–Bignami disease, a rare alcoholic demyelination of the corpus collosum, presents with subacute impairment of higher mental function accompanied by clouding of consciousness, ataxia and epilepsy.

Dementia: Chronic Organic Brain Syndromes

About 5% of individuals over the age of 65 years suffer from dementia in moderate or severe form, the prevalence rising to over 20% in the over 80 year-olds. Sufferers are amongst the most difficult patients, and for relatives and carers the demented patient produces great psychological demands. Not only does the patient suffer loss of memory but usually also a marked change in personality to the extent that a wife may say that "the man to whom I've been married for 40 years is no longer there; I am looking after a different person".

The management of patients suffering from dementia and the support of their relatives is outside the general scope of this book and reference should be made to texts listed at the end.

Senile Dementia of the Alzheimer Type (SDAT)

This is the commonest type of dementia and probably affects two thirds of patients with a dementing illness. Alzheimer's disease is usually subdivided into two types.

Alzheimer's disease type 1 (AD1) characteristically develops in individuals over the age of 75 years and has a more benign course with a slow decline in cognitive function. Alzheimer's disease type 2 (AD2) arises before 75 years of age and has a more rapid progression. In AD1 the main deficit is in cognition, typically with dysphasia and memory impairment, the patient exhibiting little in the way of motor dysfunction; life expectancy may be little affected in this condition. In AD2 the cognitive decline is commonly accompanied by evidence of other cortical dysfunctions, including agnosia, dyspraxias and visuo-spatial disorders. These patients commonly show alterations in motor function, particularly affecting gait and postural stability, and epilepsy. Patients with AD2 have a reduced life expectancy, most dying before the age of 80 years.

The typical history of memory impairment in Alzheimer's disease is of a gradual downhill course without any obvious sudden or stepwise deterioration. In the early stages the memory loss may be attributed to the minimal forgetfulness of the elderly. The onset may be so insidious that it is difficult for the patient's family and friends to pinpoint exactly when it began, and in many cases they may not even realise that the patient has anything wrong other than "old age". The patient may be found to be dementing only when she reaches the stage at which her behaviour becomes disturbed, difficult to cope with or obviously dangerous, and breakdown of the social situation has occurred. The dementia may also first be diagnosed if the patient presents to medical services with some other (usually physical) condition and is noticed to be forgetful or is found to be so on formal testing of memory.

The memory loss in the early stages is mainly for recent events and testing of short-term recall highlights this problem. The patient often seems perplexed by her situation and surroundings. As the disease progresses the patient more obviously also loses the ability to recall events which occurred long ago. There is commonly disorientation in time, place and person, the last being distressing to family and friends who may no longer be recognised. Agitation and depression are common but psychotic features are rare. Some patients may develop disinhibition (loss of social "control" which may manifest as aggression, abnormal sexual advances, swearing uncharacteristically and the passing of urine and faeces in inappropriate situations), dysphasia, dyspraxia, and agnosia. Motor function may also be abnormal with the development of extrapyramidal features such as rigidity, gait disorder and akinesia. Extensor plantars are common.

In the later stages of the disease disturbed behaviour may be particularly prominent with shouting, aggression, incontinence and faecal smearing. The management of such patients can be extremely difficult and it is often at this stage that the psychogeriatrician first becomes involved. For many patients with dementia earlier involvement of the psychogeriatrician in assessment and management offers anticipation of future problems, counselling of relatives and the setting up of supportive networks which achieve much in ameliorating some of the later effects of the disease.

In the final stages the patient may be withdrawn, mute and unresponsive. She is likely to be completely immobile and will sit in a chair or lie in bed all day without complaint. She gives no indication that she wishes to go to the toilet and may be unable to co-operate with nursing, requiring to be dressed and fed. Pre-terminally rapid weight loss is often seen.

The Vascular (Arteriosclerotic or Multi-infarct) Dementias

Dementia due to vascular disease is the next commonest cause of dementia after Alzheimer's disease. It is likely that in most cases it results from the accumulation of cerebral infarcts secondary to arterial embolism from extracerebral sites including the carotid circulation and, perhaps, in some cases the heart. Though originally thought to be a well-defined entity it is now apparent that dementia due to vascular disease has been diagnosed in life more frequently than can be accounted for by subsequent neurohistological findings.

There are probably several reasons for this, including the occurrence of other types of dementia which exhibit fluctuations in severity from time to time and the incidental co-existence of cerebrovascular disease with senile dementia. In the latter case the diagnosis of vascular dementia may be made when a patient suffering with early senile dementia has a minor cerebral infarction (such infarctions being relatively common in the elderly) which produces clinical evidence of focal neurological abnormality.

The neurohistological changes in patients with vascular dementias take a variety of forms. Some patients have diffuse areas of infarction throughout the cerebrum whereas others have small numbers of larger infarcts. Areas of lacunar softening may be found in the cortex, subcortex or both. A rarer form of vascular dementia is due to diffuse subcortical white matter demyelination and is known variously as subcortical arteriosclerotic encephalopathy, chronic subcortical leucoencephalopathy or Binswanger's disease. In this condition CT scan shows periventricular white matter translucency, especially in the frontal white matter. Binswanger's disease tends to present between the ages of 50 and 70 years, most patients having a history of hypertension. Half of the patients present with acute neurological deficit and are then found to be demented. The dementia is commonly insidious, progressing slowly to global intellectual impairment. The dementia is often less incapacitating than the motor features such as disorders of gait, dysarthria and pseudobulbar palsy. The focal neurological deficits commonly progress subacutely and then stabilise for long periods of time.

The overall pattern of vascular dementia is, however, of a stepwise decline in cognitive function often accompanied by evidence of motor dysfunction with lateralising signs typical of stroke. The onset is frequently acute and many cases come to attention when a typical stroke has occurred. If the onset is more gradual, emotional and personality changes and complaints of dizziness, headache and syncope may precede obvious cognitive impairment. Sudden decline in cognitive, motor, sensory and visual function occur as a result of new episodes of cerebral infarction. Relatives and friends may give a clear history of the patient suddenly "going off" and getting better over the course of several days. In the earlier stages there is restoration of function between episodes of infarction though careful testing may show that the patient never quite returns to her previous level of function. As the disease progresses neurological and cognitive deficits accumulate and the degree of recovery between episodes diminishes. The patient is eventually left with a permanent deficit.

Cognitive impairment may fluctuate considerably even from day to day or at different times in the day. Thus an acute confusional state may become particularly obvious in the evening and cause disturbance of the ward or household.

Other evidence of cerebral cortical dysfunction may be found, the motor disorder often being prominent, with generalised hyper-reflexia, hypertonia, and spasticity of gait. Emotional incontinence (laughing and crying inappropriately and without apparent control) may be seen and should not be confused with psychiatric depression or emotional lability. Emotional incontinence is untreatable whereas depression even in the context of dementia may respond well to antidepressant medication.

In vascular dementia the patient may be more aware of her disability and be able to describe times when she is muddled and times when she improves. The

Table 3.6. Hachinski ischaemic score (Hachinski et al. 1975)

If the patient with cognitive impairment shows any of the following features, score as indicated:

	Score
Abrupt onset of cognitive impairment	2
Stepwise deterioration in cognitive ability	1
Fluctuating course in cognitive impairment	2
Nocturnal confusion	1
Relative preservation of personality	1
Depression	1
Somatic complaints	1
Emotional incontinence	1
History of presence of hypertension	1
History of stroke	2
Evidence of associated arteriosclerosis	1
Focal neurological symptoms	2
Focal neurological signs	2
Total score	

A score of 4 or below suggests "primary degenerative dementia" (i.e. SDAT).
A score of 7 or above suggests "multi-infarct dementia".

degree of insight of patients with this condition is said, in the early stages, to be greater than that of patients with Alzheimer's disease. The retention of insight has been suggested as the cause of depression so often found in patients with this disorder.

The so-called "Hachinski" score has been widely used as a means of distinguishing between vascular and senile dementia (Table 3.6). The score was originally devised with relatively young and mildly affected patients and its suitability for very elderly and more severely demented patients remains in doubt. It may, nevertheless, be useful in research to separate patients with the two types of dementia and if used in conjunction with other features of the disease may assist in the diagnosis of individual patients.

There is little evidence that active intervention modifies the course of the disease. As it is probably a variant of stroke disease some clinicians look for evidence of cerebral embolism and infarction (usually by means of a CT scan) as a cause of the condition. Patients with infarction who do not have atrial fibrillation may be treated with a low dose of aspirin (75 mg daily) in an attempt to prevent progression. Those with atrial fibrillation may be considered for anticoagulant therapy but the benefits are unproven and treatment may be fraught with difficulties and dangers in patients who are already forgetful and whose compliance with medication, if not supervised, is poor.

"Reversible Dementias"

It has long been recognised that alteration in cognitive function may be found in the context of other, potentially treatable medical conditions. These changes have been observed in, for example, hypothyroidism, vitamin B_{12} deficiency, normal pressure hydrocephalus and subdural haematoma. The cognitive impairment has been referred to as "reversible dementia", the hope being that with the treatment of the causal disease the abnormality in the mental state will be reversed. It seems likely that in most cases of this type it is incorrect to call the alteration in mental function a dementia. Many of the cases described in the literature have been diagnosed as having dementia without the proper criteria having been applied. Most of these patients were probably suffering from subacute confusional states or focal brain disorder rather than with a true dementia syndrome and these conditions may be associated with treatable or reversible causes of brain dysfunction.

Subcortical Dementia

This syndrome was first defined in patients with progressive supranuclear palsy (Steele–Richardson syndrome). The patient characteristically thinks slowly, taking a long time to answer questions: so long that the doctor may mistake the failure to answer as evidence of cognitive impairment. But if sufficient time is given, the patient may give a correct answer. The patient may also show difficulty in using new information given to her, and also have a change in personality and mood. The patient lacks any features suggestive of cortical involvement (dysphasia, apraxia and agnosia).

Parkinson's Disease and Dementia

There has been debate for many years as to whether patients with Parkinson's disease and dementia have co-existing Alzheimer's disease or a dementia specific to Parkinson's disease. Recent work indicates that many of these patients have Lewy bodies, not only in the substantia nigra but also in the cerebral cortex. The condition has been given the neuropathological name of Diffuse Lewy Body Disease but the clinical syndrome is probably better named Senile Parkinsonism. Some patients with this condition present with the motor features of Parkinson's disease and later develop evidence of dementia, while others present with a cognitive deficit before motor features appear. In the early stages the dementia may be "subcortical" in type with marked slowing of response to questions rather than gross memory loss. The memory loss also shows fluctuation from time to time. As the disease progresses these fluctuations become less apparent and the memory loss more severe.

In some series of elderly patients 30% of those with "Parkinson's disease" have been found to have dementia. The majority of such patients probably have senile parkinsonism of the diffuse Lewy body type. In the past, many patients with this condition were diagnosed as having Alzheimer's disease associated with Parkinson's disease (see Chap. 8), but when these conditions do co-exist the tempo of progression is often different between the extrapyramidal features and the cognitive changes.

Dementia of Frontal Type

This is an increasingly recognised form of dementia which hitherto may have been included with cases of Pick's disease. The onset of symptoms is with personality change characteristic of impairment of frontal lobe function. There is flattening of emotional responses, with tactless and irresponsible behaviour. Mild disinhibition is frequently seen and the patient loses insight into her own behavioural changes and impairment. These features are reminiscent of syphilitic general paralysis of the insane that was seen commonly in the last century.

Memory deficit is mild, and late in appearance. Dysphasia, agnosia and dyspractic features are absent, in striking contrast to Alzheimer's disease. In a proportion of these cases muscular wasting, weakness and fasciculation complicates the disease and is indistinguishable from motor neurone disease. It generally heralds a very poor prognosis. Some patients may develop the amyotrophy first and are then diagnosed as motor neurone disease, the dementia later complicating their illness.

Normal Pressure Hydrocephalus

Because this is a potentially reversible condition it is much sought for in demented patients, but the results of shunting procedures in patients diagnosed as normal pressure hydrocephalus has, in general, been disappointing.

The classical features are the triad of mental impairment, gait disturbance and urinary incontinence. The mental state in these patients is characterised by memory loss, though in many patients there are features of "subcortical dementia" with marked slowing of cognition and psychomotor retardation. In some patients delirium may be superimposed or may indeed comprise the change in mental function. Some patients may present with other psychiatric syndromes such as depressive psychosis and have no evidence of cognitive impairment. Gait disturbance may occur at an early stage and may be the presenting feature. When the gait disturbance is mild the patient may shuffle slowly along with a broad-based gait. Falls are common and the patient may have particular difficulties in turning around. In more severely affected cases the patient may exhibit spasticity of the legs with increased knee and ankle jerks and extensor plantar responses. Urinary incontinence may be an early feature, much earlier than would be expected in patients with other forms of cognitive impairment.

This condition is rare unless there is a past history of meningitis or subarachnoid haemorrhage. Assessment for a shunting procedure is something that requires the most careful and comprehensive neurological work-up.

Pseudodementia

The term pseudodementia describes patients who exhibit features of cognitive impairment in the context of other, usually affective, functional psychiatric disorders. The original view was that the affective disorder itself produces the cognitive deficit and that the latter was, therefore, treatable. In many cases this is probably true, though more recent research has suggested that a higher than expected proportion of patients presenting with pseudodementia will develop a true dementia syndrome in ensuing years. Thus pseudodementia may represent the affective response of the brain in the very early stages of dementia, before the latter affects cognitive function to any observable extent. The underlying affective disorder is most commonly depression, but it must be remembered that depression may co-exist with dementia. This can make the diagnosis of the pseudodementia syndrome extremely difficult.

There are two main modes of presentation. The patient may be very withdrawn, inaccessible, have little coherent speech, will reject food and drink and be apparently disorientated, but show little in the way of obvious affective features. Other patients may present with agitation or apparent delirium but have no evidence of the clouding of consciousness seen in true acute and subacute organic brain syndromes.

If this presentation of affective disorder is to be detected, a very careful history must be taken. The time course of the illness and its mode of onset should be established. A short history of cognitive deficit in the context of life events that might be expected to precipitate a depressive illness should raise suspicion of pseudodementia. In some patients the presentation may occur as an anniversary event related to psychological trauma, loss or bereavement some years before, perhaps triggered by a more recent problem such as physical illness. A previous or family history of depression should be sought. The patient with pseudodementia may complain of the memory deficit which, though such a complaint may occur in the early stages of vascular dementia, is in contrast to the lack of insight in demented patients who have reached the same level of behavioural disturbance. When allowed to describe her illness the patient with pseudodementia may give a clear account of the current illness and her past life in response to open-ended questions, but replies "I don't know" to direct questions, and seems to want not to be bothered, whereas the demented patient usually tries to do her best despite getting things wrong.

Even after careful psychiatric examination the diagnosis may remain in doubt and ultimately be made as a result of ongoing observation. Often observation by nursing staff provides the evidence of depression. The patient may transiently emerge from the withdrawn or agitated state and make comments more consistent with a depressive state – for example, about her unworthiness. For some patients a therapeutic trial of antidepressants may be necessary.

An awareness of pseudodementia is very important – it is a potentially treatable state. Early involvement of a psychogeriatrician is advisable for rapid diagnosis and treatment. Careful watch should be kept on the patient's fluid and electrolyte balance and her nutritional state. Failure to do so may lead to superimposed organic confusion which may be diagnostically confusing, and potentially fatal. It may also alter her response to therapeutic measures aimed at the affective disorder.

4 Disturbances of Gait and Balance, and Falls

Falls and complaints of postural unsteadiness are commonplace in the elderly. They represent one of the major modes of presentation for a variety of illnesses, but the appropriate management and prognosis depends entirely on correct diagnosis.

Population-based studies have shown that in the younger elderly (aged 65–75 years) females tend to fall approximately twice as frequently as males. This sex difference declines amongst those aged over 75 years. In both sexes there is a steady increase in the incidence of falling until in those aged 85 years or over 45%–50% of individuals will have a serious fall in any one year. Falling is the cause of increasing morbidity and mortality from limb bone fractures and their complications (especially fractured neck of femur and pulmonary embolism). Also, by virtue of the loss of confidence experienced by "fallers" (even those who do not suffer serious injury) falls may lead to progressive limitation of day-to-day activities.

Falls may result from a wide variety of causes both neurological and non-neurological, acting singly or in combination. In some individuals, environmental factors are the most important, but with increasing age medical causes become increasingly common and disorders of the nervous system underlie the majority. Neurological disturbance of balance and gait can be classified according to the main system that is defective. Thus our knowledge and understanding of labyrinthine disorders causing vertigo is relatively comprehensive. Diseases causing weakness (either of a lower or upper motor neurone type) can be well understood to cause the classical disturbances of gait and balance that will be discussed shortly; and, similarly, sensory or cerebellar ataxia can be diagnosed following the appropriate neurological examination. But the elderly patient whose family describes her as becoming increasingly "doddery" is commonplace but seldom discussed in terms of pathology, causation, physical signs, investigation, treatment or prognosis. In this chapter we will discuss briefly those forms of gait disturbance, imbalance and falling which are due to well-defined neurological disorder – hemiplegia, paraparesis, Parkinson's disease, cerebellar ataxia, sensory ataxia, lower motor neurone weakness and episodic vertigo. But particular emphasis will be placed on that group of patients who do not "fit into" any of these categories and where osteoarthritis of hips and knees, and cervical spondylotic change does not seem adequate to explain the gross dyspractic disorder of gait and balance that is the cause of so much disability in the elderly. Attacks of loss or disturbance of consciousness may, of course, present as falling and it is always important to establish from the outset whether a patient is falling because she had a blackout, whether the fall was simply accidental tripping or whether there is a continuing disturbance of gait or balance. Attacks with disturbance of consciousness are discussed in Chapter 9.

Maintenance of Posture and the Effects of Age and Age-related Disease

The maintenance of posture is dependent on a complex system involving sensory afferents, central processing and "set" and motor components of the nervous system, together with all parts of the musculo-skeletal system. Age and age-related disease can affect any of the components involved in postural control. Although a combination of factors frequently summate to affect balance and walking there is usually one critical abnormality and it is this that must attract the major therapeutic effort. The prospects for independence and mobility depend on this assessment and treatment.

Sensory

The main sensory inputs for the control of posture are proprioceptive, visual and vestibular. Though gross abnormality of proprioception is not commonly found at examination of the elderly it is likely that the quality of proprioceptive information being relayed to the central processing systems deteriorates with increasing age. Proprioceptive information relayed from mechanoreceptors in and around joints in the cervical spine are probably of particular importance and provide information about the spatial relationships between the head and trunk. The numbers of such receptors decrease with increasing age and this loss seems to be accelerated in individuals suffering with arthritic diseases (in particular rheumatoid disease and cervical spondylosis): this loss of receptors may lead to a reduction in information from the cervical spine. It has even been suggested that in some patients this reduction in proprioceptive information is responsible for the symptoms commonly ascribed to vertebro-basilar insufficiency, rather than an abnormality of blood flow in the posterior cerebral circulation. In addition to these age-related changes, diseases such as sensory neuropathies and conditions associated with abnormal proprioception become more common with old age.

Elderly people tend to have more problems with vision than the young. Accommodation is lost so its role in assessing distances of perceived objects is impaired: if stereoscopic vision is maintained this loss can probably be overcome, but if there is a marked asymmetry in vision between the two eyes, for example, reduced visual acuity in one eye, then stereoscopic function may be lost unless the asymmetry can be rectified by appropriate refractory correction. A particular example of the problem can arise following unilateral cataract extraction when the difference in retinal image size between the two eyes may cause marked unsteadiness. This is usually overcome in time. Visual clues, important in the control of balance, may be reduced if visual acuity is diminished by refractive errors, cataracts, or retinal disease.

Diseases causing abnormalities of the vestibular apparatus should be separated into those which are episodic and those which are persistent. But the characteristic symptom of disorder of the vestibular system is vertigo.

Vertigo is defined as a "hallucination of movement". The room feels as if it is tilting or turning. Patients have to be questioned carefully before dizziness is attributed to vertigo because it is a difficult symptom to describe; and other causes of imbalance are too readily accepted as vertigo if a direct question is put – "does it feel as if everything is spinning?" – and an affirmative answer given.

Damage to the vestibular apparatus through trauma or vascular occlusion may cause acute vertigo with prostration and gross disorder of balance. The lateral medullary syndrome where a vertebral artery occlusion causes acute damage to the vestibular nuclei on one side is, perhaps, the best example. But the vertigo and imbalance usually recovers to a substantial degree as does that resulting from more minor vascular occlusions affecting the brainstem or inner ear, or those resulting from trauma. Damage to the labyrinth from poorly controlled use of aminoglycoside antibiotics may lead to a more persistent vertigo and imbalance. The episodic vertigo which results from Ménières disease, vertebro-basilar ischaemia, or the syndrome of benign positional vertigo, usually causes considerable distress and disability because each episode of symptoms is too short-lived to allow adaptation. Thus in Ménières disease the patient is struck down by an attack of vertigo lasting usually between one and four hours and causing vomiting and prostration from which it may take several days to recover. And the dread of a further attack may lead to profound psychological disturbance. Anti-emetic drugs and vasodilators probably have greater value as placebos helping to improve the patient's confidence than in any specific pharmacological effect. The unilateral deafness and tinnitus characteristic of Ménières disease persists between attacks of vertigo. But deafness and tinnitus are so common in the elderly (although usually bilateral) that diagnosis may be difficult and require assessment with otological tests.

Benign positional vertigo is a disorder of vestibular function characterised by intense vertigo provoked by rapid change of head position. It may be caused by head injury, or may follow viral illness or a small vascular occlusion. When a patient describes symptoms suggestive of benign positional vertigo specific clinical tests should be performed as follows.

The patient is sat upright on the couch. The headrest is lowered and pillows are removed. The patient is told that the examiner wants to assess whether dizziness can be provoked by head movement and that she will, therefore, be asked to lie back quickly with her head turned to one side: and to keep the eyes open. The examiner then holds the patient's head and lies her back quickly, simultaneously turning the head to one side. Two observations are then made. Does the patient complain of dizziness and indicate distress? Does the patient develop nystagmus?

Patients with benign positional vertigo develop dizziness and nystagmus 5 to 15 seconds after change of head position and the effect wanes within 60 seconds.

In the majority of cases of benign positional vertigo no cause is discoverable and a diagnosis of acute labyrinthitis is offered. It has been suggested that this condition results from a disturbance of the otolith apparatus on one side, by dislocation or damage to the hair cells. Whatever the pathology, recovery is the rule, over a time scale of many months. During this time the patient must be advised to avoid sudden head movement and, therefore, to take especial care looking for the traffic when crossing the road or when reaching to pick something off the floor.

A single isolated incident of vertigo and loss of balance with no decrement of hearing is generally attributed to "vestibular neuronitis". Recovery generally takes place over a period of a few weeks.

Phenothiazine anti-emetics should always be used with the greatest care. In general their therapeutic effect in the vertiginous patient is disappointing whereas the side effects can be serious. These side effects include sedation, depression, parkinsonism, postural hypotension, constipation and hypothermia. (Acute dystonic reactions are rare in the elderly.) Occasionally they may provoke the serious persisting phenomenon of tardive dyskinesia.

It seems likely that the three sensory systems – proprioceptive, visual and vestibular – are complementary in function and tend to back up each other. This is certainly the case for vision. Thus, when postural stability is studied by measurement of anterior-posterior sway over a set period of time, the amount a subject sways is significantly greater when the eyes are closed than when they are open. In the elderly this complementary role of the three sensory systems may be particularly important; if one system is functioning poorly the other two may be able to compensate for the deficit in the first; if all three systems are limited in the information they provide then, for example, a decrease in visual acuity produced by poor environmental illumination may be sufficient to produce loss of postural control and a fall. This summation of factors producing dizziness is sometimes referred to as the Multiple Sensory Dizziness Syndrome (MSDS).

Elderly people tend to stoop and look downwards when they are walking, because of an age-related change in central "set" of posture, and degenerative or osteoporotic changes in the spine. This posture leads to a reduction in information about horizontals and verticals, and striking improvement in steadiness of gait may be achieved if the patient can be encouraged to look ahead.

Motor

The motor system is complicated in that movement is produced and co-ordinated by a number of different systems, most importantly the pyramidal, extrapyramidal and cerebellar systems acting together. Any of these systems can be affected by ageing and age-related disease.

Stroke with hemiparesis, or paraparesis from spinal cord compression affects the descending pyramidal pathways with the characteristic unilateral or bilateral disturbance of gait and balance. The patient complaining of falls, or disturbance of balance from these causes seldom presents any difficulty in diagnosis because the physical signs of an upper motor neurone lesion are easily elicited (weakness, increased tendon jerks, spastic hypertonia without wasting of muscle, and extensor plantar responses). The posture of the hemiplegic is characteristic – with flexion of the upper limb and extension of the lower limb giving foot drop and circumduction of the foot during walking. Similarly, the patient with paraparesis may be easily diagnosed by the stiff-legged gait and tendency to tilt the trunk in order to lift the spastic foot drop clear of the ground.

Parkinson's disease (see Chap. 8) may be difficult to distinguish from hemiplegia as a cause of gait disturbance, especially when the extrapyramidal features do not include tremor and are unilateral. But the signs of rigid (as opposed to spastic) hypertonia, bradykinesia and absence of weakness should serve to make the distinction.

The loss of Purkinje cells from the cerebellar cortex is one of the most clearly established age-related cell losses in the central nervous system. As the cerebellum is concerned with the co-ordination of movement and balance it seems likely that this loss of cells has effects on stability. The cerebellum and its connections are frequently affected in vascular disorders of the brain. Most types of cerebellar degeneration present before old age, but examples are seen of late onset hereditary and non-hereditary cerebellar degeneration. Cerebellar degeneration due to thyroid disease is a reversible condition and must always be considered. Cerebellar degeneration may occur as a non-metastatic manifestation of a malignancy, especially carcinoma of the bronchus or gynaecological cancers. Toxic damage to the cerebellum may result from alcohol and occasionally anticonvulsants (especially phenytoin) or sedatives. Unfortunately if toxic exposure has been present for more than 3 weeks, there is seldom complete recovery.

Patients with these mid-line (vermis) degenerative disorders of the cerebellum usually have early and severe disturbance of balance and gait, reminiscent of drunkenness and associated with dysarthria. In contrast, cases of damage to the cerebellar hemispheres, for example from vertebro-basilar stroke, show nystagmus and limb ataxia with inco-ordination.

Musculo-skeletal Changes

Muscle strength decreases with age and there is evidence that the loss accelerates in later decades: between the ages of 20 and 60 years a total of about 7% of muscle strength is lost, whereas in those over 60 years of age the rate increases and about 7% is lost each decade. Undoubtedly age-related changes occur in striated muscle, loss of fast fibres being particularly marked. The exact mechanism for this age-related loss is unclear, but it is likely that whole motor units are lost either through motor neurone degeneration in the spinal cord or degeneration in some motor fibres in peripheral nerve. Decreased physical activity also results in loss of muscle power. Some inactivity in the elderly is related to altered social roles and perceptions after retirement, but some is undoubtedly due to limitations imposed by physical disease; for example, pain in the legs which is particularly common in women. Conversely, increase in physical activity as a result of altered lifestyle and the relief of symptoms such as pain offers the possibility of increased muscle power with benefit in the stability of large weight-bearing joints such as the knee and hip.

Neuropathies

The neuropathies seen commonly in old age are those due to diabetes, carcinoma and alcohol. Dysproteinaemic neuropathy (including myeloma), toxic and nutritional neuropathies and, occasionally, Guillain–Barré syndrome are other rarer causes. The symptoms and signs are similar to those found in younger patients. Postural unsteadiness results from a combination of factors – loss of peripheral tactile information, loss of proprioception and joint position sense, and decrease in motor power due to involvement of motor nerves in the pathological process. The patient with alcoholic neuropathy usually has a typical polyneuropathy with muscular pain and tenderness, or burning in the feet with tremor of the hands.

Subacute Combined Degeneration of the Cord

Vitamin B_{12} deficiency due to pernicious anaemia becomes increasingly common in old age. The condition was called "subacute" because progression from first symptoms to major disability may occur in weeks. Early diagnosis and treatment is, therefore, important and a serum B_{12} estimation should always be done in any patient with any of the features of this condition, that is, peripheral neuropathy, paraparesis or proprioceptive loss. Occasionally patients are seen with the classical neurological signs of subacute combined degeneration of the cord with little in the way of anaemia or macrocytosis but who, nevertheless, have a subnormal serum vitamin B_{12} level. The diagnosis of the condition on clinical grounds may be made difficult by the alteration in some neurological signs with age: vibration sense is frequently found to be absent below the knees in otherwise normal individuals; testing of joint position sense in the feet may be difficult in the patient with cognitive impairment.

The treatment of elderly patients with a profound degree of anaemia (below 8 g/dl) with injections of vitamin B_{12} may suddenly increase haemopoiesis and lead to hypokalaemia, consequent cardiac dysrhythmias and even death.

Potassium supplements are advisable in such patients (providing of course there is no hyperkalaemia prior to therapy as a result of coexisting renal failure) together with careful monitoring of serum potassium levels.

Gait Dyspraxia

Many patients with progressive acquired gait disturbance, loss of balance and falling will be found not to fit into any of the categories described above.

Thus the history will contain no mention of vertigo or attacks of disturbance of consciousness. The patient shows no weakness of the limbs sufficient to explain her difficulty in walking. There are few signs of hemiplegia, cerebellar disturbance, or sensory loss. But in spite of this absence of the classical clinical features of neurological deficit the patient needs assistance to stand or walk or may already have deteriorated to the point where she is wheelchair-bound.

In the absence of objective abnormality to explain disability of this degree, psychological factors may be invoked. But it is very rare in the elderly for a primarily psychological disturbance to affect solely gait and balance. Patients with severe depression may take to their chair or bed but this behaviour is characterised by the mood of depressive withdrawal and retardation.

It is commonplace in the very elderly for the patient to report that when sitting she feels steady and free from any sense of weakness, loss of balance or sensation. But as soon as she attempts to stand the sense of balance is clearly defective. The patient may lean so far backwards when she attempts to stand that she has to be supported. Or she may only be able to remain on her feet if holding onto the furniture or a frame.

When the patient starts to walk the co-ordination required to move the body weight onto one foot in order to advance the other is obviously lacking. Start hesitancy where the feet seem frozen to the floor with "marche a petits pas" (characteristic of parkinsonian gait) is typical and is usually a very striking feature of this disorder. Posture may be flexed (again as in Parkinson's disease) but is more often rather erect and upright. The patient reports a sensation of extreme instability amounting to a conviction that she will fall unless she is supported either by hanging on to something secure or by being helped. But the feeling of instability is immediately relieved by sitting down.

Gait dyspraxia probably results from any condition causing dysfunction in the frontal lobes including the motor association areas. It is also seen commonly in patients with senile parkinsonism where it was described vividly by James Parkinson himself. But it is important to distinguish gait dyspraxia due to parkinsonism from other causes because in Parkinson's disease there is usually some response to dopamine agonists (See chap. 8) whereas in other disorders there is no response to these agents.

The specific clinical diagnosis seldom leads to specific therapy but the management in terms of occupational therapy, appliances, physiotherapy and, above all, prognosis is determined by the natural history of the underlying disorder. Patients of any age who present with gait dyspraxia should be carefully assessed and investigated. Loss of locomotion in the elderly rapidly becomes a self-perpetuating phenomenon so that the too-early provision of aids such as a wheelchair may lead to irreversible deterioration. By contrast, skilled physiotherapy may achieve remarkable improvement in walking ability. Where the family can maintain the motivation and confidence required to walk, this improvement can often be maintained with enormous benefit in independence.

Parkinson's disease is discussed in detail in Chapter 8. There is a temptation to diagnose any patient presenting with the disturbance of balance and gait characteristic of gait dyspraxia as a case of Parkinson's disease, but there are good reasons for resisting this temptation and trying to achieve a definitive diagnosis.

Thus a therapeutic trial of dopamine agonists seldom resolves the diagnostic dilemma. These agents tend to exacerbate cognitive disturbance and provoke hallucinosis. And some patients with senile parkinsonism (diffuse cortical Lewy body disease) show only a poor therapeutic response to these agents.

Similarly the natural history of Parkinson's disease is different from that of the other conditions listed in Table 4.1 and causing gait dyspraxia.

The diagnosis of these conditions depends on clinical features that serve to distinguish them from Parkinson's disease. Alzheimer's disease is characterised by early and steadily progressive cognitive disturbance which may be remarkably focal initially (causing dysphasia, or spatial disorientation) and is usually associated with memory impairment. These features will normally be clearly established by the time Alzheimer's changes have led to gait or balance disturbances so that Alzheimer's disease is unlikely to be the diagnosis in the absence of serious memory impairment.

A stroke affecting the frontal lobe may be "silent" clinically or cause hemiparesis from which recovery is complete. But a second stroke on the other side may produce disproportionate disability with severe balance disturbance and gait dyspraxia. Furthermore, recovery from the effects of a double hemiplegia from multiple infarcts is often disappointing.

Diffuse cortical Lewy body disease is responsible for senile parkinsonism in a substantial proportion of elderly patients. The clinical features and treatment of this condition are fully dealt with in Chapter 8.

Binswanger's encephalopathy or subcortical arteriosclerotic encephalopathy is a condition where progressive dementia is associated with neurological

Table 4.1. Causes of gait dyspraxia

Parkinson's disease
Alzheimer's disease
Multi-infarct disease
Diffuse cortical Lewy-body disease
Binswanger's encephalopathy (subcortical arteriosclerotic encephalopathy)
Frontal space-occupying lesion (metastases, subfrontal meningioma, glioma)
Normal pressure hydrocephalus
Traumatic (boxers) encephalopathy
Multi-system atrophies
GPI (general paralysis of the insane)

symptoms and signs, hypertension and frontal periventricular white matter changes on CT scan (which is not seen in multi-infarct dementia). The neurological signs are typically those of gait and balance disturbance associated with pyramidal and extrapyramidal signs and normally with some degree of dementia. Similar clinical features are seen in patients in whom both frontal lobes are affected by metastases, bilateral subdural haematoma or empyema, subfrontal meningioma or other primary tumour and also in cases of normal pressure hydrocephalus. These conditions can usually be diagnosed on the basis of the clinical features and the CT scan appearances. Thus normal pressure hydrocephalus may be suspected where ventricular enlargement is associated with little or no evidence of atrophic change over the convexity of the brain.

Multi-system atrophy tends to present in middle life and is relatively rare in the old or very old. The clinical features are those of parkinsonism (with gait dyspraxia), autonomic failure (particularly postural hypotension) and cerebellar signs. This is a slowly progressive disorder in which atrophy of one of the systems may predominate. Thus severe parkinsonism with slight orthostatic hypotension may give a clinical picture difficult or impossible to distinguish from Parkinson's disease. And the effects of dopamine agonists in causing postural hypotension may lead to further diagnostic and therapeutic problems. The disease responds poorly to levo-dopa and the course is slowly progressive.

General Paralysis of the Insane (GPI). A short case history probably best illustrates GPI as a cause of gait and balance disturbance.

Case 4.1
A 68-year-old man was admitted to a major postgraduate teaching institution for investigation and treatment of progressive ataxia of gait. He was thought to have signs indicative of cerebellar degeneration but CT scan showed no features of this whereas marked frontal atrophy was noted. A variety of diagnoses were offered by the several neurologists who saw him but the correct diagnosis was only made when routine serological testing reported a positive Wasserman reaction.

Treatment

The physiology of gait dyspraxia is poorly understood but probably depends on damage to frontal motor association areas concerned with the learnt "programme" for walking and control of balance. Experience confirms that treatment by pharmacological means has little effect on gait dyspraxia, except in Parkinson's disease where dopamine agonists in adequate dose may have a specific and curative effect. In all the other disorders discussed in this chapter, physiotherapy is the only effective form of treatment. These patients must be discouraged from taking to a wheelchair. A programme should be established of daily or twice daily walking and balancing exercises. Emphasis must be placed on building up the patient's self-confidence because the experience of injury from one or more falls has usually led to a situation where the patient dare not attempt to learn again to stand and walk.

Appliances and aids to walking have an important place in the treatment of gait dyspraxia. Whereas patients with musculo-skeletal disorders or sensory ataxia may benefit from the use of a standard Zimmer frame, patients with gait dyspraxia seldom find this appliance helpful. Their difficulty is to maintain their own balance sufficiently to lift the Zimmer frame and move it forward. "Wheeled-walkers", especially those which are reasonably robust and are provided with a braking system, provide the optimal appliance for most patients.

5 Headache and Facial Neuralgia

At all ages headache is a common symptom. Because popular belief has it that headache commonly indicates the presence of brain tumour (which of course it does not) and because brain scanning has been associated in the public mind with the successful treatment of brain tumour (which, sadly, is untrue) patients present with headache often and with the unspoken but implicit request for a CT scan. There must be a temptation for the doctor to dispose of the problem by requesting a scan without diagnosing the cause of the patient's headache. Not only is this bad medical practice but it is unsatisfactory and occasionally dangerous: unsatisfactory because it leaves the patient reassured that he has a normal scan but still with his symptom and the potential for deterioration due to an undiagnosed cause and dangerous because not only are there many serious causes of headache that give a normal scan but also because the CT scan can miss brain tumour, subdural haematoma and a host of other structural intracranial disorders.

In the elderly, facial neuralgias are more common than in the young, so that a knowledge of this group of disorders is essential in geriatric practice. Headache is no less common in the elderly than in the young, but headache arising de novo in an old person has a greater significance than in the young or middle-aged. Elderly patients presenting with headache seldom have a psychoneurotic basis for their symptom; and migraine in all its variants has a tendency to improve with increasing age.

The diagnosis of headache or neuralgias usually depends on two things, the recognition of a pattern of symptoms characteristic of a known disorder and the discovery or exclusion of specific physical signs. The history is, therefore, all-important but it may be difficult. An old person, in pain, is likely to be impatient for relief and disinclined to co-operate with exhaustive questioning from a doctor. Patients will always emphasise the severity of the pain, but this feature is among the least helpful in diagnosis. The doctor needs information about duration, distribution and quality of the pain (whether it is sharp, aching, burning, or like pins and needles). Above all he needs to know the pattern of the symptom – whether it is episodic or continuous and, if episodic, whether the attacks last moments, minutes, or hours. He needs to know all the associated symptoms – catarrh, scalp tenderness, visual disturbance or loss of balance. And finally he needs to know what provokes and what relieves the symptom. A patient in severe continuous pain will be accompanied or surrounded by anxious relatives who are likely to be more insistent that the doctor "do something" than keen to answer questions about duration of the headache and preceding or associated changes in the patient's behaviour.

It is, therefore, essential that the doctor can approach the subject with a classification of the causes of headache or neuralgia and a knowledge of their essential clinical features and treatment. A therapeutic trial of treatment for this complaint seldom solves a diagnostic dilemma – more commonly the reverse. Thus it is commonplace to see a patient who has been taking carbamazepine for months – or longer – because she told her doctor that it "seemed to help" her facial pain due to temporo-mandibular arthropathy or sinus pathology.

Headache

Chronic headache due to benign conditions like migraine or tension headache is less common in the old than earlier in life. Patients with chronic headache tend not to present in old age – they have "learnt to live with" the problem and are secure in the knowledge that their long-standing headache is benign. Headache presenting for the first time in old age must, therefore, always be taken seriously.

It is useful to classify the causes of headache into two groups. Extracranial headache includes those conditions giving rise to headache which affect structures outside the skull (or within the bone as in the case of Paget's disease or bone tumours) and where the physical signs are generally localised in the head. Intracranial headache includes conditions giving rise to headache but arising within the skull where physical signs are exclusively neurological.

Extracranial causes for headache are commoner than intracranial ones, and also generally easier to detect on careful physical examination. Intracranial causes of headache are more often due to vascular occlusion or subdural haematoma than to tumours. Thus cerebral tumour usually presents with epilepsy or progressive loss of focal brain function with or without signs of raised intracranial pressure; and in the old, raised intracranial pressure is often not accompanied by headache.

Extracranial Headache

Cranial Arteritis
There are few conditions where the correct diagnosis leads to such dramatic and gratifying response to treatment or where failure to diagnose may lead to such disaster. This diagnosis must always be in the forefront, in any elderly patient presenting with headache (and occasionally other symptoms, as discussed elsewhere).

Case 5.1
An 83-year-old male had fallen, suffering brief concussion. Thereafter he complained of severe headaches, was unwell with weight loss and became withdrawn. Scan was normal. Because subdural haematoma had been excluded no diagnosis was made until two months later when his ESR was found to be 94. Rapid recovery occurred on treatment with steroids.

The typical story is of gradually worsening headache which is generalised and aching in quality. The pain may be confined to one part of the scalp or spread into the back or front of the neck or into the face – for example, the orbit, jaw or tongue. Pain in the jaw muscles or tongue may be exacerbated by chewing due to arterial insufficiency. There is often associated tenderness noticed by the patient when she brushes or washes her hair or rests her head against the pillow. The patient will usually admit to general symptoms of ill-health such as weight loss, lack of energy, fever, vague aching in the back or joints and loss of appetite. Examination will usually, but not always, reveal some tenderness of the scalp or neck. The temporal arteries or their branches may be thickened with redness of the overlying skin, and these and the occipital or facial arteries may be non-pulsatile.

Wherever cranial arteritis is suspected, an immediate ESR should be taken and the patient asked to wait until the result is known. While typically the ESR will be substantially raised, occasionally there is only modest elevation of the ESR. If the diagnosis is likely then immediate steroid treatment should be begun, with prednisolone 40 mg daily reducing slowly. Within 48 hours the patient will be recovering from her headache and feeling dramatically better. There is, of course, no response to steroids in symptoms caused by the ischaemia from occluded vessels and this may account for the continuing headache in some cases.

Some doubt about the diagnosis of temporal arteritis will arise where the ESR is only slightly raised or, in the less common situation, where the symptoms are atypical but the ESR very high, as might happen for example in myeloma. Biopsy of a cranial vessel may be helpful in this situation, but care must be taken to choose a vessel that is tender and hence likely to show the diagnostic giant cell changes. Biopsy may also be indicated if there is a high risk of side effects from steroid treatment (e.g., a patient with diabetes or severe hypertension). A negative biopsy result does not exclude the diagnosis so that the evolution of the symptoms and signs may still indicate treatment with steroids.

The patient is only out of danger from vascular occlusion after she has been on treatment with steroids for several days, but no additional treatment (e.g., anti-coagulants) seems to affect the outcome if blindness or stroke supervene. The ESR falls rapidly as soon as steroid treatment is begun (in contrast to most cases where the ESR is raised for other reasons) and headache ceases to be a problem. Thereafter headache is a poor guide to the effectiveness of maintenance steroid therapy. This should be judged by serial ESR measurements so that the patient continues on an alternate day steroid dose at the lowest dose level required to keep the ESR below 20. Prednisolone treatment may have to be continued for long periods of time and the author has seen two cases who

suffered major stroke and blindness respectively following withdrawal of steroids in the presence of an ESR in the 20s after 2 and 4 years of continuous
steroid treatment.

Herpes zoster

There are few more humiliating experiences for the hospital specialist than to be
rung up by a relative to say that the patient with headache he saw yesterday and
could not diagnose has now developed a rash on one side of his forehead.
Herpes zoster typically presents with severe head pain in the 10%–15% of
shingles cases where the condition affects the first division of the trigeminal
nerve. The pain may precede the rash by as much as a week. It is resistant to
analgesics and in the old it may be difficult to obtain a clear account of the
unilateral and predominantly frontal distribution of the headache. Similarly,
examination may not easily demonstrate sensory loss in the appropriate area
and a reduced corneal reflex unless these signs are specifically and carefully
looked for. As soon as the rash develops the diagnosis can be made by the
patient. Treatment with oral acyclovir accelerates recovery from the skin lesions
and associated pain but does not seem to affect the incidence or severity of
post-herpetic neuralgia. Steroids administered within 48 hours of the onset may
reduce the incidence of post-herpetic neuralgia.

Ramsay–Hunt syndrome or *Herpes zoster* oticus (also idiopathic Bell's palsy)
may present with headache, localised usually behind the ear. The pain may
precede the facial palsy by up to a week.

Sinus pain and Headache from ENT or Dental Conditions

Infection or neoplasia as well as conditions altering the pressure in the
para-nasal sinuses may all give rise to headache or facial pain. The localisation
of pain from ENT or dental causes tends to be referred to the territory of the
cutaneous innervation of the nerve involved. Thus pain of nasal origin tends to
be referred to the orbit or cheek on the affected side (maxillary nerve) whereas
pain from ear conditions is perceived over the back of the scalp immediately
behind the ear (C2) or deep in the ear (Xn). Increased sinus pressure is not
apparently painful in the experimental subject but "vacuum headache" from
occlusion of the ostium of a nasal sinus gives rise to a constant localised
unilateral pain over the sinus and increased by local pressure – for example, on
the cheek (maxillary sinus) or beneath the inner superior margin of the orbit
(frontal sinus). In ethmoidal sinusitis pain is typically over the bridge of the nose
and may be associated with tenderness of the eyeball.

When catarrhal symptoms accompany lateralised headaches as described,
diagnosis may be relatively straightforward but it is usual for ENT examination
to be necessary with appropriate X-ray examination for a definite diagnosis
and, above all, in the elderly for the exclusion of neoplasia. However, in cases of
sphenoidal sinusitis, vertex or frontal headache may be associated with ophthalmoplegia, or ophthalmic division trigeminal sensory loss due to involvement of
the superior orbital fissure and must be distinguished by appropriate imaging
from other cavernous sinus syndromes. Neoplasia involving the maxillary sinus
often involves the maxillary nerve far enough back in the sinus to cause

anaesthesia not only of the cheek but also the upper jaw and hard palate (middle superior alveolar nerve).

Arthropathy

Pain from arthritis or degenerative changes of the temporo-mandibular joints or cervical spine may present as diffuse headache lacking the clear relationship to posture or movement that characterises joint pain elsewhere.

Temporo-mandibular arthropathy (Costen's syndrome) gives unilateral pain, which may be widespread over the side of the face and head. It is typically an episodic pain lasting hours and may develop following dental extractions or injury to the side of the face. The bouts of headache are typically after chewing, e.g., a steak, but occasionally the pain is present on waking when it is worth enquiring of the spouse whether the patient habitually grinds his teeth during sleep. There may be some degree of trismus on examination but most characteristically the joint is tender and crepitus can often be demonstrated.

Considering the fact that degenerative changes in the cervical spine are practically universal in the elderly it is remarkable how rarely these changes give rise to pain, either localised in the neck or referred to the head. It is important to bear this in mind and not jump too readily to the conclusion that headache is due to cervical spondylosis. It is also important not to accept too readily a diagnosis of cervical spondylotic headache made by another doctor on the basis of X-ray film changes. Whiplash injury of the neck may be followed (often after an interval of several days) by head and neck pain thought to be derived from changes in the apophyseal joints of the upper cervical spine. The pain is associated with restriction of neck movement and tends to be exacerbated by certain postures such as leaning over a desk or driving for long periods.

The occipital neuralgias are a group of headaches where posterior unilateral pain results from a disorder of the greater occipital nerve. In the elderly, paroxysmal occipital neuralgia is not uncommon. It is experienced as lancinating spasms of pain over the back of the head, occasionally triggered by pressure over the upper neck muscles or by movements of the neck. There is no sensory loss or other physical sign, and treatment with carbamazepine will usually suppress the neuralgia until spontaneous remission occurs. Continuous occipital neuralgia or "posterior cephalgia" may be caused by lesions of the foramen magnum or posterior fossa. There must be careful examination for upper cervical or posterior fossa neurological deficit and appropriate radiological investigation must be pursued if abnormal neurological signs are found. But occasionally continuous occipital pain presents without signs of central neurological disorder and with tenderness over the greater occipital nerve, and dysaesthesia of the posterior scalp. This condition is probably an irritation of the posterior occipital nerve at the C1/2 joint and, while difficult to treat, is generally benign and self-limiting.

Rheumatoid arthritis of the cervical spine tends to involve the atlanto-axial joint, leading to subluxation at this joint. Occipital headache aggravated by neck flexion is the most common symptom. Any patient with rheumatoid arthritis complaining of headache should be investigated with appropriate X-ray examination for atlanto-axial joint subluxation.

Bone Pain

The skull vault should be palpated in patients with headache, especially the elderly, because benign and malignant tumours of bone as well as Paget's disease may present with headache.

Paget's disease of the skull may be obvious from the facial appearance but often the deformity of the skull can only be detected by palpation and even then there may be uncertainty. An X-ray examination of the skull in undiagnosed headache is fully justified to exclude Paget's disease as well as conditions such as pituitary lesions, sphenoid ridge meningioma or metastatic skull deposits. Paget's disease may cause cranial neuropathies, especially deafness, and occasionally progresses to malignant osteogenic sarcoma of the skull.

Of the benign tumours invading bone, meningioma is the commonest in the head but occasionally osteoid osteoma or venous bone cysts may be seen and their removal relieve the patient of her symptoms. Metastatic lesions of bone or malignancies such as myeloma or osteosarcoma are fortunately rare. But the base of the skull is not uncommonly invaded by neoplasm arising in the nasal cavity or pituitary region.

Migraine

It is relatively unusual to see migraine presenting over the age of 65 years. When it does it should be investigated with the same diligence as is applied to epilepsy of late onset. Thus it should be assumed until proved otherwise that migraine of late onset is symptomatic of some intra- or extracranial vascular disorder. Head injury may provoke typical migraine headaches in the elderly and these tend to be persistent. Hypertension may present in this way. And anaemia, or respiratory failure, are the causes of headache which often follows a "migrainous" pattern. Vascular intracranial tumours or vascular occlusion as causes for migraine headache will be considered later.

Paroxysmal hypertension from phaechromocytoma may present with very severe usually posterior headaches lasting usually 10–15 minutes. They may be accompanied by pallor, palpitations and a sense of anxiety reminiscent of a panic attack.

Intracranial Headache

Not all the intracranial structures are pain-sensitive, so that brain tissue itself is not sensitive to pain nor is the convexity dura away from the venous sinuses. But the Circle of Willis and the main cerebral and cerebellar arteries for 1–2cm, the venous sinuses, the IInd, Vth, IXth, Xth and XIth cranial nerves and the dura over the base of the skull are sensitive to pain. The basal meninges and main arteries in the anterior and middle cranial fossae are innervated by the trigeminal nerve, so that there is a tendency for pain derived from these structures to be referred frontally; whereas the posterior fossa and contents are supplied by the glossopharyngeal nerve and tend to be referred occipitally. Lateralisation of the pathology from the side of the headache is usually reliable.

Stroke

Cerebro-vascular disease is an important and common cause of headache, but little emphasis is given to this symptom in standard texts. This leads, for example, to the mistaken belief that a patient with hemiplegia and headache probably has a brain tumour. It also leads to failure to diagnose cerebral vascular disease or even to consider the possibility when typical headache is unaccompanied by the appropriate neurological deficit.

Case 4.2

A 74-year-old male presented with the complaint of moderately severe right orbital pain which had come on during the night and persisted severely for the 6 days before he was seen. There were no associated symptoms and the pain was partly relieved by analgesics.

On examination he had slight constriction of the right pupil with minimal ptosis, and a bruit over the right carotid bifurcation. There were no other eye signs nor any sign of hemisphere disturbance. Carotid angiography showed complete occlusion of the right internal carotid artery.

Occlusion of the internal carotid artery commonly causes headache referred to the ipsilateral orbit or eyebrow. In completed stroke the pain is persistent, usually resolving over a period of weeks but occasionally going on indefinitely. Transient ischaemic attacks (TIAs) may cause episodic headache, clearing in minutes or hours and mimicking "migraine of late onset". The pain is usually attributed either to inflammatory changes in the wall of the artery or to painful dilatation of anastomotic channels. This latter mechanism probably accounts for the more persistent headaches after stroke.

Headache is less common in middle cerebral artery occlusions than it is where the internal carotid artery is involved, but the pain tends to be perceived in the orbit, frontal or temporal regions on the side of the occlusion. Posterior cerebral artery occlusions give rise to headache that is usually localised to the frontal region on the same side, but in the lateral medullary syndrome with vertebral artery occlusion the headache is occipital or nuchal.

Stroke from intracerebral haemorrhage is commonly associated with headache related to displacement of the brain or mid-line structures, raised intracranial pressure and leakage into the subarachnoid space. Pituitary apoplexy where haemorrhagic infarction of the pituitary causes ophthalmoplegia, amblyopia and acute pituitary failure is characteristically associated at onset with severe central frontal headache.

Aneurysms

The headache of an aneurysm *per se* is commonly not diagnosed until after rupture has occurred. Following subarachnoid haemorrhage a history may be obtained of headache, probably from the aneurysm. But the headache of the subarachnoid haemorrhage itself is usually dramatic. There is sudden severe lateralised headache, which quickly becomes generalised and associated with neck stiffness and vomiting. In the absence of brainstem or lateralising neurological signs or signs of raised intracranial pressure the diagnosis is confirmed by lumbar puncture. The pain of subarachnoid haemorrhage exceeds that of all other intracranial catastrophes. In the elderly aneurysm presenting as subarachnoid haemorrhage carries a very poor prognosis.

Aneurysms may present in other ways especially in the old. They may present as a space-occupying lesion causing headache, facial neuralgia, or fits. Posterior communicating artery aneurysm may present with orbital pain, ophthalmoplegia and trigeminal sensory loss and paraesthesiae in the ophthalmic division. Or they may present as an incidental finding on plain X-ray examination (when the aneurysm is calcified) or CT scan. The assessment and management of aneurysm is a neurosurgical matter, but in the elderly conservative management with symptomatic treatment is usually preferable.

Chronic Subdural Haematoma (CSDH)

The CT scan has proved a reliable method of diagnosing chronic subdural haematoma although occasionally an isodense or bilateral haematoma can still be missed. But the clinical indications for scanning for CSDH are difficult. The clinical diagnosis may be overlooked where there is no clear history of trauma and the symptoms and signs are non-specific. The prognosis following surgery in the elderly patient is much less satisfactory than generally believed. Clinicians are fearful of criticism for failing to diagnose the CSDH which is found at post mortem – the implication being that the haematoma arose solely as the result of minor trauma and could be cured by surgical evacuation. Neither supposition is likely to be correct.

Although a history of trauma to the head is usual in CSDH, occasionally no such history can be obtained. CSDH has resulted from lumbar puncture, epilepsy (without apparent head injury) and commonly where there are disorders of blood coagulation (particularly excessive alcohol consumption). An almost invariable symptom in CSDH, however, is headache. Any patient with headache, insidious and fluctuating neurological deterioration and a history of head trauma or the predisposing features described should be investigated for CSDH by CT scan.

The demonstration of CSDH does not necessarily indicate that neurosurgical treatment is appropriate. In the elderly, evacuation of the haematoma is commonly followed by failure to improve, a chronic low pressure state with often the recurrence of subdural haematoma on the same or opposite side.

When a CSDH is diagnosed in a patient making an uncomplicated recovery from head injury it is usually preferable not to intervene but to follow the spontaneous resolution of the haematoma by CT scan. A large symptomatic haematoma should probably be evacuated, although this decision will be influenced by the age of the patient, the degree of pre-existing cerebral atrophy and a history of alcoholism, or clotting disorders. In patients over the age of 70 years, CSDH carries a relatively poor prognosis and is not the benign condition often suggested in the older textbooks.

Space-occupying Lesions

In the elderly patient it is not uncommon to see a massive cerebral tumour present late and with only recent onset of headache. It is generally assumed that the normal atrophic changes in the brain leave more room within the cranial cavity for space-occupying lesions to expand before intracranial pressure rises. The features of raised intracranial pressure are the same at all ages – generalised morning headache, vomiting, progressing to visual failure from the effects of the pressure on the optic nerve. In the elderly gait disturbance, confusion and incontinence are often prominent additional non-specific features of rising intracranial pressure and may mimic the features of the adult hydrocephalus syndrome. Papilloedema is less frequently seen in this age group, even where there is massive space occupation within the skull.

Pituitary tumours may present in old age when the signs of hypopituitarism or acromegaly may be more difficult to discern than in early life. Presenting symptoms often include a mild variable confusional state, bitemporal headache and a lethargy often attributed to old age. The critical signs are visual field defect, typically bitemporal, with pallor of the optic discs. The transphenoidal surgical approach to these tumours is relatively well tolerated even in frail individuals.

Meningioma typically presents in the second half of life and is the commonest intracranial tumour in the old. It must be diagnosed on the basis of clinical suspicion in the context of features suggesting a progressive mass lesion. It is probably true that before CT scan many operable meningiomas in the elderly were not diagnosed. Now it is more common for the surgeon to be faced with the dilemma of whether an elderly patient with an operable meningioma or other benign tumour will withstand the trauma of neurosurgery and make a useful recovery within a reasonable time span. A recent review from Detroit (Dujovny 1987) has, however, reported an operative mortality of only 2% in a series of patients over 65 years.

Psychogenic Headache

In early or middle life headache is more frequently the result of anxiety states than depressive illness. In the old the reverse seems to be true. "Involutional" depression often developing in the context of illness or injury is commonly associated with symptoms of headache. The diurnal mood swing with the symptoms maximal in the morning may suggest the possibility of raised intra-cranial pressure but careful questioning will usually elicit the fact that the headache is not present on waking but develops after the patient has woken up.

Tension headaches, when they occur in the elderly, are also more common as a symptom of an agitated depressive state. Restless depressive rumination about constant head pain and its sinister significance may be relieved rapidly and in a most gratifying manner by a course of treatment with antidepressant drugs. By contrast, reassurance seems to be a less potent therapeutic weapon in this age group and the elderly tend to be less impressed and reassured by the trappings of "high tech" medicine such as CT scan.

A chronic involutional hypochondriasis, often with headache as a major symptom is a more intractable problem. Antidepressants are unhelpful and sedative drugs generally contra-indicated. Phenothiazines or haloperidol are probably the most useful drug treatment and some success has been achieved with pimozide or sulpiride. But the possibility of causing tardive dyskinesia indicates caution in this therapeutic approach.

Facial Neuralgia

Not all facial pain in the elderly is due to trigeminal neuralgia. While this statement is obvious, it is remarkable how often a diagnosis of trigeminal neuralgia is put forward because no alternative suggests itself in spite of there being none of the clinical features of the condition. As with headache, diagnosis is the essential basis for investigation and treatment: and diagnosis depends on a detailed history as well as the relevant examination against a background of knowledge of the differential diagnosis. "Neuralgia" here will be taken to imply any facial pain, whatever its duration, because it is the patient presenting with facial pain in the outpatient clinic that we have in mind. However, the paroxysmal neuralgias of cranial nerves V and IX (and possibly X) have features in common that distinguish them from other neuralgic facial pains attributable to migrainous, psychological or local causes.

Trigeminal Neuralgia

Trigeminal neuralgia has an average age at onset of 50 years but since the condition is benign and requires continuing supervision, cases accumulate in geriatric practice. In the majority the condition is "idiopathic", that is unassociated with any discoverable causative pathology; but rarely trigeminal neuralgia may develop as part of multiple sclerosis, posterior fossa tumour (especially in the cerebello-pontine angle), Paget's disease or following lateral medullary syndrome. In these secondary cases abnormal physical signs are usually present, particularly nystagmus and sensory loss in the face, whereas in idiopathic trigeminal neuralgia physical examination should not reveal any neurological deficit except possibly minimal subjective sensory disturbance.

The diagnostic features of the condition are pain that has the following characteristics. It is unilateral and confined to the trigeminal territory (i.e., does not cross the mid-line or extend behind the ear onto the neck or back of the head); It is severe, paroxysmal and is triggered by more than one type of local stimulus (a single stimulus such as biting or talking may indicate a local painful lesion in the mouth). With trigeminal neuralgia two or more triggers are necessary for diagnosis – such as swallowing and washing the face. Trigeminal neuralgia may rarely develop bilaterally but when it does the paroxysms of pain are independent of each other. Similarly it may occur in association with the other cranial nerve neuralgias, especially glossopharyngeal neuralgia. The pain is often localised, at least to begin with, to one division of the trigeminal nerve and the mandibular division is the most commonly involved. The paroxysmal characteristics of the pain are important. It is an intense pain for brief moments of time repeated so frequently that the pains become almost continuous. Typically patients with trigeminal neuralgia go through bouts when for weeks or months the pain recurs frequently either spontaneously or by being triggered. And then there is remission also for weeks or months followed by another bout. Not all patients enjoy remission and in this case medical treatment may have to be continued at high dosage indefinitely. The pain is so severe that no patient can be expected to put up with it. Trigeminal neuralgia is a medical emergency that needs urgent assessment and treatment.

Carbamazepine is the medical treatment of choice for this condition. It is more acceptable, better tolerated, has fewer complications and is more reliably effective than surgical treatment. It is, therefore, strange that many doctors and patients believe that surgery or trigeminal injection is the only proper cure. When carbamazepine is ineffective at maximum tolerated dose or when intolerable side effects develop (especially skin rashes) trigeminal nerve injection is nearly always necessary because drugs other than carbamazepine seldom have any significant effect (phenytoin, clonazepam or baclofen can be tried). Carbamazepine should normally be started at a dose of 100 mg three times daily and increased every 48 hours until pain control is achieved, up to the maximum tolerated dose, usually 1200–1400 mg daily. When the patient has been free from pain for 4 weeks slow reduction of dose by decrements of 100 mg each week may allow complete withdrawal of treatment. If a maintenance dose is not necessary to keep the patient pain-free she should nonetheless be advised to keep a small supply of carbamazepine available for the day when the neuralgia recurs.

The surgical treatment of trigeminal neuralgia can be separated into three alternative approaches.

1. The most effective form of treatment with least trauma to the patient is ganglion or root thermocoagulation or radio-frequency lesion. Early relief of pain can usually be achieved in over 90% of patients but recurrence of pain may occur in about 10% within two years. The risks of the procedure are of damage to adjacent cranial nerves or the carotid artery. Modern techniques involve trigeminal nerve stimulation before the lesion is placed and in this way a high proportion of cases may enjoy dissociated pain relief with preservation of light touch. However, occasionally dense sensory loss in the face may result from this form of lesioning and lead on to keratitis or ulceration of the skin of the face or mucous membranes. In a small proportion of cases intractable causalgic pain develops in the affected trigeminal territory and resists all forms of treatment.

2. Peripheral neurectomy or nerve injection is a simple and relatively safe procedure of particular value where the mandibular division alone is affected in the very elderly or frail individual.

The supra- and infra-orbital nerves can be injected in appropriate cases, but this technique suffers the disadvantage of giving only temporary relief with recurrence of pain usually within 12 months.

Glossopharyngeal neuralgia may be surgically treated by peripheral nerve neurectomy or avulsion and here the frequency of recurrence of symptoms is less than it is in trigeminal neuralgia.

3. Posterior fossa microvascular decompression has been pioneered by Jannetta. It involves a craniotomy and carries a 2% risk of serious complication. Recurrence of pain occurs within 6 months in some 15% of cases and Janetta himself has commented "I am in . . . a dilemma about recommending microvascular decompression . . . because the procedure must be carefully learned if the surgeon is to avoid unnecessary morbidity and mortality".

Post-herpetic Neuralgia

This condition gives no problems of diagnosis but the problems of successful treatment are formidable. Post-herpetic neuralgia in the elderly tends to be a cause of severe pain and dysaesthesiae resistant to all forms of treatment. It generally develops gradually while the herpetic skin lesions are healing and then continues with gradual improvement over a time scale of some 18 months in the more fortunate cases. Sensory impairment in the affected area can always be demonstrated and is associated with painful hypersensitivity of the skin. The pain is continuous but often waxes and wanes according to the patient's mental or physical state. Thus stress or physical fatigue tend to exacerbate the pain, and it is tolerated best if the patient is mentally and physically occupied.

Post-herpetic neuralgia involving the head or face is unsuitable for treatment with transcutaneous electrical stimulation, which some patients find helpful elsewhere. Antidepressants in full dosage (e.g., imipramine) combined with an anticonvulsant such as valproate or carbamazepine is the most reliably effective form of treatment, but frequently this pain proves resistant to all therapy. There is no place for surgical destructive procedures.

Migrainous Syndromes

Migrainous neuralgia and lower facial migraine are rare conditions overall. They are very rare in the elderly. But occasionally facial pain having the characteristic features of cluster headache, facial migraine, or chronic paroxysmal hemicrania may be seen in the old. These conditions should be considered where no local cause for facial pain can be found and where the symptoms do not fulfil other diagnostic criteria.

Atypical Facial Pain

Chronic intractable localised or general facial pain may be the presenting symptom of depressive illness. The history is often complicated with preceding episodes likely to be migrainous, or due to tension headaches. The development of continuous aching pain in the face, accompanied by overt or covert depressive symptoms, characterises the admittedly somewhat vague entity of atypical facial pain. But this condition is worthy of recognition, because it usually responds satisfactorily to antidepressant treatment when it has proved resistant to all other means of therapy. Tricyclic antidepressants are usually effective in full dosage although mono amine oxidase inhibitors may occasionally be necessary.

6 Some Visual Problems

Patients with visual disturbance usually present with vague non-specific symptoms. "Blurring" of vision may be symptomatic of anything from monocular blindness to bitemporal hemianopia; or from vertical diplopia to oscillopsia; or from refractory error to impaired colour vision. Even highly intelligent individuals seem to have difficulty in analysing the nature of their visual disturbance and it is commonplace for hemianopic field defects to be mistaken for monocular visual disturbance. When the symptoms are transient and leave behind no abnormal physical signs diagnostic uncertainty may be inevitable.

In the elderly, visual disturbance is frequently multi-factorial. At the very least, some degree of presbyopia will normally complicate a visual problem. And opacities of the media with cataract and additional retinal, corneal or pupillary disorders may add to the difficulties. In this chapter consideration will not be given to primarily ophthalmic conditions – iritis, corneal disorders, abnormalities of the lens or glaucoma.

The examination of the optic and oculomotor nerves in the elderly patient may pose particular problems. The fundi may be difficult to see for a number of reasons. Elderly patients often have difficulty in keeping their eyes fixed and are intolerant of the bright light of the ophthalmoscope. The pupil tends to be smaller in old age than in the young. And the media may be opacified. It is sometimes difficult to hold the attention of an elderly person sufficiently to examine eye movement adequately and, particularly, where there is double vision the patient may not tolerate exhaustive tests of this type. Conjugate upward gaze is normally reduced in old age and the same applies to convergence of the eyes. Fatiguable nystagmus may be demonstrable on full lateral gaze, especially if the fixation target is held less than one metre from the subject. This sign is without significance.

Visual acuity should always be tested with the patient wearing the appropriate spectacles (distance glasses when using the Snellen chart; reading glasses when using the Jaeger type – but ensure the glasses are clean. The Snellen chart gives a more reliable and reproducible test of visual acuity). When testing visual acuity it is important to be aware of the possibility that the patient's difficulty may be due to a specific reading difficulty or visual agnosia. Following stroke, patients with defects of this type may present with symptoms of difficulty reading without any associated neurological deficit to provide the clue. An 'E' test where the patient is asked to orientate a hand-held letter E to match a Snellen series of variously orientated letters may be the most suitable method of testing acuity in such a case.

Where there is double vision care must be taken to observe for any unilateral displacement of the globe of the eye. Minor degrees of Horner's syndrome can be easily overlooked and may be important in the diagnosis of internal carotid artery pathology.

Visual failure is usually a symptom that holds particular dread for the old person. It signals loss of independence of degree greater than that from loss of any other sense or through inability to walk. Great importance must be attached to emphasising the reassuring aspects of the prognosis and careful explanation of the mechanism for the visual symptoms and the prospects for treatment must always be given.

Neuro-ophthalmological problems presenting in old age fall into a number of separate groups. Thus there are the episodic or paroxysmal disorders, particularly those related to transient disturbances of ocular or cerebral arterial perfusion and, by way of contrast, those disorders of vision that are persistent or progressive. These may be separated into those disturbances of the visual pathways behind the chiasm and those that are pre-chiasmal. And, finally, there are the neurological disorders (and they are mostly neurological) which give rise to double vision.

Episodic Visual Disturbance

Amaurosis Fugax

Transient monocular visual disturbance (Amaurosis fugax) is due to embolisation of the central retinal artery and is probably the commonest example of a *transient ischaemic attack*. The patient notices a sudden painless loss of vision in one eye "like a shutter or curtain coming down". The embolus may occlude all arterial perfusion to the retina or it may block a branch retinal artery causing transient altitudinal hemianopia. The visual loss normally recovers within 5 minutes and frequently in less than 1 minute, as the embolus breaks up and is carried through the capillary circulation. Patients giving this history should always be questioned about transient or persisting symptoms suggestive of contralateral hemiparesis or hemianaesthesia – indicative of cerebral embolisation from the same source. Smoking, diabetes, polycythaemia, hyperlipidaemia and hypertension are all predisposing factors and must be carefully investigated. Occasionally amaurosis fugax may be mistaken for migraine or even acute glaucoma. In subsequent management it becomes important to distinguish between emboli arising in the heart and those arising in the carotid artery.

Embolisation from the heart may occur in patients with cardiac dysrrhythmia, especially auricular fibrillation, rheumatic heart disease and recent myocardial infarction and in patients who have had cardiac valve replacement surgery. It is generally accepted that all patients in this group should remain on anticoagulant treatment indefinitely unless there is major contra-indication. Bacterial endocarditis, myxoma, or calcification and incompetence of the mitral valve may also provide a source for emboli and require appropriate medical or surgical treatment. These conditions must always be borne in mind in any patient presenting in this way.

Emboli arising in the carotid artery are more common than those from the heart and there is greater dispute about appropriate management. Treatment must be assessed against the evidence from Framingham, Massachusetts that 30%–40% of patients with transient cerebral or retinal ischaemic attacks suffer stroke or death from myocardial infarction within 3 years. Aspirin is probably the most effective treatment, at least in men, in reducing the incidence of stroke. The optimal dose is uncertain but 150–300 mg daily is a generally recommended regime. Treatment should probably be continued indefinitely. Other drugs known to reduce platelet aggregates in vitro and, by extrapolation, emboli in vivo (sulphinpyrazone, dipyridamole) have not been shown to reduce the frequency of amaurotic attacks nor the incidence of stroke.

Emboli from the carotid artery may be associated with an identifiable bruit most commonly at the carotid bifurcation and angiography may confirm a stenosis or plaque of atheroma providing a source for embolism. The appropriate treatment strategy for lesions of this type is at present uncertain. Anticoagulants, fibrinolysins, surgical endarterectomy and angioplasty are all currently being evaluated.

Occasionally, embolisation from the carotid results from trauma to the artery – either a direct blow or penetrating wound or stretching of the vessel as in a whiplash injury. Anticoagulant treatment with heparin is indicated in this situation.

Embolisation affecting the posterior cerebral artery or arteries may cause a different type of transient visual disturbance. If the occipital cortex is rendered ischaemic, transient homonomous hemianopia will occur. Occasionally emboli divide at the bifurcation of the basilar artery and simultaneous bilateral striate cortex ischaemia results. In this situation the symptom is one of complete transient blindness of a cortical type.

Impairment of retinal perfusion as the result of stenosis or occlusion of major arteries in the neck without embolisation may lead to intermittent symptoms of monocular blindness, field defect or distortion of vision. Signs of retinal ischaemia may be detectable on fundoscopic examination but usually require fluorescein angiography for confirmation. Typically the visual symptoms are provoked by standing up from sitting or lying.

Angiography of the major cerebral vessels will allow assessment for vascular surgery in suitable cases.

Migraine

Episodic visual disturbance may be the result of classical migraine attacks. Where such symptoms present after the age of 60 years they should always be viewed with suspicion. Like the focal epilepsies, migraine of late onset may indicate a vascular cerebral tumour.

The important diagnostic feature of migraine is that the visual disturbance *evolves*. The patient typically describes a paracentral scotoma; this is usually perceived as a shimmering blind spot which starts as a blob and then, over a period of minutes, evolves into a crescent, often with an irregular coloured margin. The crescent gradually moves towards the periphery of the visual field on one side and finally disappears after 20–30 minutes. Any one part of the visual field tends to be involved for a few minutes so that the original scotoma recovers normal vision as the crescent is extending. The headache that follows the visual disturbance may be asymmetrical and range from very severe to non-existent.

It is now believed that the migrainous process is an electrical one – the spreading depression of electrical potential in the cortex first described by Leao – possibly with secondary changes in scalp and brain perfusion. Classical migraine, as described, may present in old age as a recurrence of a migrainous tendency from early life (primary classical migraine). It may also develop as the result of severe hypertension, cerebral embolism especially in the posterior cerebral territory, cerebral tumours in the occipital lobe especially very vascular lesions, or occasionally as a late manifestation of a long-standing arterio-venous malformation.

Symptomatic treatment of primary classical migraine in the elderly is with simple analgesia – soluble aspirin or paracetamol – taken at the onset of symptoms when its absorption can be achieved before the headache is established. Ergotamine tartrate is more liable to side effects and is also less well tolerated in old age. Continuous prophylaxis is rarely required but beta-blockers such as propranolol are occasionally useful for this purpose.

Epilepsy

The occipital lobe is peculiarly resistant to epileptic phenomena; and the temporal lobe only rarely gives rise to episodic visual disturbance as an aura to an epileptic seizure.

Epilepsy is, therefore, only an occasional cause of disturbance of vision. But explosive visual symptoms with bright coloured lights "like fireworks" may occur as an aura to a major fit: or as a focal partial epileptic phenomenon, where it is usually easily clinically distinguishable from TIA by the positive visual features (bright coloured lights or spots or lines) and from migraine by the short duration of the symptoms and their failure to evolve and move slowly over the visual field. Like migraine, epilepsy of this type suggests a focal structural disturbance of the brain and should be investigated with CT scan.

Persistent and Progressive Visual Disturbance

Prechiasmal (and Retrobulbar) Lesions

Persisting visual symptoms resulting from primary optic neuritis are rare after the age of 60 years. The great majority of patients, therefore, who present with the complaint of pain and failing vision in one eye, and where the cause is retrobulbar with no detectable abnormality in the eye itself, will have either a vascular pathology affecting the optic nerve or optic nerve compression. Where the symptoms are simultaneously bilateral, toxic causes (tobacco, alcohol and certain drugs) and general systemic diseases have to be considered.

Ischaemic optic neuropathy presents with the sudden onset of visual loss affecting all or part of the field of vision in one eye. The optic disc looks pale, swollen and the distinctive clinical feature is the narrowing (by comparison with the veins) of the arteries of the retina. There may be linear haemorrhages at the disc margin. Cranial arteritis (see Chap. 5) is an important cause, but embolism, polycythaemia or other blood disorders and atheroma may present in this way. Vasculitis of the retinal or choroidal vessels may complicate *Herpes zoster*, polyarteritis or possibly sinusitis. The prognosis for recovery of vision in these cases is very poor. If the second eye becomes involved at a later stage the features are of unilateral disc swelling with contralateral optic atrophy or "pseudo-Foster–Kennedy Syndrome" (see below).

Progressive visual impairment usually suggests a compressive lesion of the optic nerve. Diagnosis may be very difficult, because there are often unrelated ophthalmic reasons for impaired vision; and serial visual field charting may be difficult, especially in the elderly. The visual acuity will be impaired with central scotoma but the fundi may be normal.

Minor degrees of displacement of the globe have great importance and significance in this context, because they usually indicate an orbital tumour. These are the province of the ophthalmic surgeon but can now be comprehensively investigated pre-operatively by scanning and angiography.

Meningioma arising in the optic canal or the inner sphenoidal ridge is the commonest compressive lesion in the elderly. Pituitary tumour, aneurysm, granuloma and rarely other neoplasms have all been recorded. Occasionally, frontal tumour may cause progressive optic atrophy on one side due to direct pressure on the optic nerve; with papilloedema on the other side from general rise of intracranial pressure (Foster–Kennedy syndrome).

While CT scanning through the orbit and lower cranial cavity will identify and define the majority of compressive lesions, X-ray examination of the optic foraminae may provide important information in, for example, the early optic nerve sheath meningioma. Radiotherapy without histological proof of the diagnosis of meningioma may be justified in the elderly patient and this form of management may lead to useful recovery of vision or at least delay of the deterioration whereas it is unfortunately the case that exploration of the optic nerve in a patient with failing vision runs high risk of immediate permanent blindness.

Chiasmal compression is less common in the elderly than in the young or middle-aged but presents greater problems of diagnosis. Acute chiasmal compression from pituitary apoplexy (haemorrhagic infarction of the pituitary) may be particularly difficult to diagnose. Early collapse and death from hypopituitarism will result unless immediate treatment is given, with hydrocortisone and measures to maintain blood pressure. These patients typically present with headache (sometimes with subarachnoid blood) ophthalmoplegia and unilateral or bitemporal visual failure. But the symptoms of collapse may make the eliciting of ophthalmic signs very difficult. Although CT scan will normally suggest the diagnosis, angiography is a wise preliminary to surgery, to exclude aneurysm.

Slowly growing pituitary tumours, suprasellar meningioma or aneurysms causing chiasmal compression usually present in the elderly with the classical features of endocrine disturbance and bitemporal field defects. But it is not uncommon at this age for these lesions to present with a variable confusional state, progressive memory disturbance or psychosis. The diagnosis should, therefore, be considered in elderly patients presenting with confusional states or dementia (see Chap. 3).

Retrochiasmal Lesions

Homonymous hemianopic visual field defects are the typical feature of a retrochiasmal lesion affecting the optic tract, optic radiation, or visual cortex. The pathology of the lesion is usually either cerebral infarction or a space-occupying lesion. The localisation of the lesion clinically is based on associated symptoms and signs of temporal lobe or parietal lobe deficit.

Any homonymous hemianopic field defect that involves the lower quadrant is a bar to driving a car. It also tends to cause considerable disability by rendering the patient clumsy in, for example, tripping over furniture or knocking over liquids at table.

Damage to the occipital cortex bilaterally causes cortical blindness with preservation of normal pupillary responses to light stimulation. The patient may deny blindness (Anton's syndrome), thereby giving rise to diagnostic difficulties with suspicion of a hysterical basis for the symptoms. Partial or complete recovery from this form of blindness is not uncommon, especially where the pathology is due to posterior cerebral artery embolism or severe hypertension rather than cranial arteritis, malignant meningitis or Jakob–Creutzfeldt disease.

Double Vision

It is useful to classify the causes of double vision on an anatomical basis provided that the two commonest causes of diplopia in the elderly are not forgotten – vascular causes and diabetes mellitus. Thus a disturbance of eye movement may be due to a primary muscle weakness, myasthenia gravis or lower motor neurone disturbance, or arise through involvement of brain stem mechanisms. The diagnosis rests on a clinical evaluation according to Table 6.1.

Ocular myopathy rarely presents in the elderly but myasthenia gravis frequently develops after the age of 60 years. Myasthenia gravis is easier to diagnose when it presents with ptosis or diplopia than when it involves only limb, bulbar, or trunk musculature. Typically myasthenia gravis affects vertical eye movement more than horizontal movements. It may be associated with thyrotoxicosis or thymoma (benign or malignant). The diagnosis is confirmed by intravenous edrophonium 10 mg ("Tensilon"). In the elderly, myasthenia gravis can be a malignant progressive condition where there is great difficulty in controlling symptoms with anticholinesterase drugs and steroids; and where the chest complications of the disease are a major cause of morbidity. The treatment of myasthenia gravis with prednisolone (which should always be introduced very slowly) has greatly improved the symptomatic control over that which can be achieved with drugs such as pyridostigmine and neostigmine. However, the complications of long-term steroid treatment in the elderly may be considerable.

The commonest causes of external ophthalmoplegia (disturbance of the lower motor neurone of the IIIrd, IVth or VIth cranial nerves) are listed in the table. In the majority of elderly patients presenting with double vision of this type, the cause will be vascular. If diabetes mellitus or cranial arteritis are excluded the prognosis for full recovery in the vascular cases is good, with the majority free of double vision within 10 weeks.

Table 6.1. Ophthalmoplegia in the elderly

Muscle: Bilateral involvement often with weakness of other muscles
   Ocular Myopathy
     ?Mitochondrial
     ?Associated with pharyngeal or facial weakness or cardiomyopathy

Myoneural junction: Vertical eye movement, ptosis, and increases on sustained muscle contraction, recovers with rest
   Myasthenia gravis

Lower motor neurone   (III, IV, VI) Follows the pattern of distribution of the cranial nerve(s) involved
   Vascular disease and cranial arteritis
   Diabetes mellitus
   Aneurysm
   Tumour, especially naso-pharyngeal carcinoma, meningioma, pituitary
   Raised intracranial pressure (VI)
   Basal meningitis, malignant tuberculosis or other (rarely) Miller–Fisher syndrome
   Paget's disease

Nuclear or supranuclear disturbences of eye movement
   Vascular disease
   Wernicke's encephalopathy
   Brainstem tumours or dorsal mid-brain metastases (Parinaud's syndrome)
   Steele–Richardson–Olszewski's syndrome
   Conjugate gaze palsy in lesions of the cerebral hemisphere

---

Progressive ophthalmoplegia requires investigation for a compressive lesion such as tumour or aneurysm. Nasopharyngeal carcinoma may be difficult to diagnose until ENT examination and biopsy under anaesthetic has been carried out. And basal meningitis diagnosed on CSF cytology may present with symptoms only of double vision.

A general rise of intracranial pressure even where there is no headache may cause an abducens palsy and present with double vision.

Guillain–Barré acute polyneuropathy may involve the brainstem, with signs of ophthalmoplegia (lower motor neurone in type) and often with cerebellar signs. This variant of acute polyneuritis is often called the Miller–Fisher syndrome and like the Guillain–Barré syndrome it carries a good prognosis.

When diseases of the central nervous system cause disorder of eye movement they generally do so by causing gaze palsy or conjugate (that is bilateral) disturbance of movement of the eyes. The commonest and most familiar example of conjugate gaze palsy (but one that does not present with visual symptoms) is the hemisphere stroke involving fronto-pontine fibres and causing the patient to be unable to look to the side of the lesion. Similarly a posteriorly situated stroke paralyses eye pursuit movements to the side of the affected parieto-occipital region. It is frequently associated with a homonymous hemianopia.

Brainstem disorders comprise a group of important diseases in the elderly. Wernicke's encephalopathy is seen in those with poor nutrition, particularly when the unsatisfactory diet is associated with excessive alcohol consumption. The disturbance of higher mental function may overshadow eye signs, especially where there is disturbance of consciousness. In these cases the diagnosis is easy to miss. (see Chap. 9).

Case 6.1
A 72-year-old female living alone was referred to hospital after her relatives had found her confused and drowsy following a short "flu-like" illness. On examination she could be roused only with difficulty and, with the poor level of co-operation, memory and eye movement could not be adequately tested although a VIth nerve palsy was queried. A plasma thiamine later showed profound deficiency and she made a dramatic recovery with thiamine injections.

In Wernicke's encephalopathy, nystagmus is common and abducens palsy (unilateral or bilateral) or horizontal gaze palsies are commoner than pupillary abnormalities or ptosis. Because this is a treatable condition, it should be considered in any elderly patient with complex ophthalmoplegia. In these cases, blood should be taken to test for thiamine levels and an immediate injection of thiamine should be given.

Brainstem stroke, or tumours affecting the brainstem, either by compression or distortion, will give a pattern of symptoms and signs often capable of precise localisation on the basis of the known neuroanatomy. Thus, in Parinaud's syndrome paralysis of conjugate upward gaze is associated with loss of convergence and pupillary abnormalities caused by a lesion affecting the corpora quadrigemina. And in Benedikt's syndrome involvement of the red nucleus and third nerve accounts for the association of an ipsilateral oculomotor palsy with a contralateral cerebellar tremor.

Steele–Richardson–Olszewski syndrome is an important and not uncommon variant of the parkinsonian syndrome. More properly called Progressive Supranuclear Palsy it presents as a tetrad of symptoms:

Akinetic/rigid parkinsonism

Early loss of vertical following eye movement (with preservation of reflex "dolls head" eye movement) with later loss of all eye movements

Personality change with loss of initiative and flattening of affect going on to dementia

Axial rigidity particularly affecting the neck and associated with a rather erect posture (in contrast to Parkinson's disease) and falls.

The disease is a progressive degenerative condition with a course from diagnosis to death of usually 3–5 years. The parkinsonian features may respond slightly to dopamine agonists (see Chap. 8) but no treatment helps the symptoms due to the disorder of eye movement, which in the early stages of this condition is often the patient's greater complaint.

Visual Hallucinations and Disorders of Visual Perception

Visual hallucinations are a common feature of the acute confusional states of the elderly. Either endogenous or exogenous toxic disturbances of the nervous system may present with complex visual hallucinations, either with or without insight. Thus, for example, a patient with cardiac failure or a urinary infection may present giving vivid descriptions of complex visual hallucinations; these may have an affective quality from which the patient may be entirely detached, or about which she merely expresses curiosity. Visual hallucinations are not usually of any localising or specific value but should be considered a common response of the elderly brain to illness, rather analogous to a fever in a younger person. (However they are a specific and prominent characteristic of delirium tremens.)

Case 6.2
A 65-year-old female with Parkinson's disease had tolerated a moderate dose of levodopa with substantial physical benefit. She then became ill with what later turned out to be a urinary infection. In addition to deteriorating in terms of her parkinsonism she also developed vivid visual hallucinations which had an obsessive quality although she did not profess to being disturbed by them. Thus every time she looked out of her window, Mrs. S.D. would see children climbing the trees in her garden and felt compelled to ask her husband to tell them to go away.

Treatment of the urinary infection allowed restoration of her necessary dose of levodopa without return of the hallucinations.

Specific disorders of visual perception may have localising value and are sometimes difficult to recognise in clinical practice. Stroke or tumour involving the parietal lobe on one or both sides of the brain may present with a visual agnosia – an inability to recognise or use objects such as spectacles, cigarette lighter or a box of matches. Prosopagnosia is an inability to identify by their facial appearance people who are familiar to the subject; and visuo-spatial agnosia is an inability to perceive the size or position of objects by vision. The patient complains of being unable to judge distance for picking up an object from a table, or the speed of traffic when crossing the road. Writing or drawing may become impossible and these visual symptoms and signs may occur in the absence of any demonstrable abnormality of the visual fields or on routine neurological examination. Visual perceptual difficulties may herald the onset of cerebral atrophy. Any patient presenting with symptoms suggesting the possibility of a visual agnosia should be asked to copy simple drawings, to construct a set pattern with matchsticks and to write a short sentence. If possible her behaviour, particularly for eating or finding her way round the ward, should be noted. Objective abnormalities indicative of any unexplained disorder of visual perception are an indication for CT scan.

7 Incontinence

Of all the neurological symptoms in the elderly, incontinence is the one most dreaded by patient and family alike. It is the symptom that changes the patient to being socially unacceptable and casts doubt on his independence and home care. Unfortunately, incontinence is one of the most common presentations of disease in old age. Many disorders, including infections, mild strokes, myocardial infarction, pulmonary emboli and heart failure come to light in this way as, of course, do disorders of the genito-urinary tract and neurological disorders affecting the frontal lobes, spinal cord or cauda equina. In most cases incontinence occurs when a specific condition arises in someone whose elimination control mechanisms are already impaired by some other disease process or by the effects of age.

Urinary incontinence is more common than faecal incontinence but, for a variety of reasons, the exact prevalence of urinary incontinence is difficult to assess. Different surveys have used different definitions of incontinence; there are problems in detection of incontinence by doctors often because the symptom is not specifically asked for as a routine in all consultations, and patients frequently will not admit to being incontinent because of the shame they feel.

Faecal incontinence is most frequently found amongst heavily dependent patients living in institutions. When found in patients living in the community, faecal incontinence is one of the factors most erosive of carers' ability to continue coping with the patient at home. Though urinary incontinence is a major problem and requires proper investigation and treatment, faecal incontinence is a medical emergency for an elderly person and requires immediate admission to hospital: to do otherwise will lead to prolonged, perhaps permanent hospitalisation, because carers find it difficult to continue caring, without help, for someone who has become faecally incontinent.

Urinary incontinence has been the subject of increasing professional interest and many health authorities have incontinence services and clinics run by collaborating geriatricians, gynaecologists and urologists, together with interested radiologists and specialist nurses. In many places where formal services are not established there are, nevertheless, specialist nurses called Nurse Continence Advisers with their own professional organisation, The Association of Nurse Continence Advisers. Continence advisers are able to provide considerable help to medical services in the diagnosis (using some of the non-invasive techniques described later in this chapter) and management of incontinent patients, and are increasingly playing a valuable educational role for other professional groups, especially nurses, within hospitals and the community.

Urinary Incontinence

Normal Control of the Bladder

The reflexes which are responsible for the control of the bladder and urinary sphincters relay in the S2 to S4 segments of the spinal cord. Sensory information about bladder filling may be derived from stretch receptors situated submucosally in the bladder wall but stretch receptors in the pelvic floor may also be important, the bladder in a sense being "weighed". The motor nerves to the bladder muscle are of the cholinergic parasympathetic type, the ganglion cells being situated in the pelvic plexus near the bladder. The internal sphincter is supplied by noradrenergic sympathetic fibres from L1 and 2. The external bladder sphincter is innervated by myelinated nerves through the pelvic plexus. The pelvic floor (piriformis, coccygeus and the levator ani), which is also important in the maintenance of continence, is innervated by S2, 3 and 4 via the pudendal nerve.

The activity of the sacral reflex arcs is modulated by cerebral cortical activity. There appears to be a cortical centre controlling micturition in the anterior part of the cingulate gyrus in the medial (parasagittal) frontal lobe. The centre is probably responsible for inhibiting spinal reflex activity when there are only small volumes of urine in the bladder, and for "social" control of micturition or the ability to inhibit bladder emptying until a convenient time and place. The descending pathway in the spinal cord is situated in the antero-lateral white matter bilaterally closely related to the spino-thalamic tracts.

The main structures responsible for continence are the integrity of the pelvic floor which, in the normal state, maintains the base of the bladder horizontal; and the trigone, which is composed of two groups of muscle fibres, those passing forwards and downwards into the urethra and those which sweep around the anterior part of the trigone and keep the internal urethral meatus closed ("the fundus ring").

Micturition is initiated by contraction of the detrusor, which leads to opening of the internal meatus and then contraction of the fundus ring leads to funnelling of the bladder neck. At the same time there is reflex relaxation of the external sphincter and descent of the pelvic floor, which passively contributes to the funnelling of the bladder neck; cessation of micturition is the reverse of this sequence.

The Effect of Ageing

There are multiple effects of ageing on the neurological control of the bladder. Loss of cortical neurones may result in a diminution of cortical inhibition of micturition, the process being enhanced in stroke disease or dementia. Such neuronal loss may affect bladder control not only directly through loss in the micturition centre but also by impairment of social awareness and memory. Little is known of the effects of age on spinal reflex arcs, nor on smooth muscle. It is not known, for example, whether there is a loss of smooth muscle within the bladder wall with age. (But, on the contrary, in outlet obstruction the bladder wall and detrusor muscle hypertrophies.) Neurogenic atrophy of the striated muscles of the pelvic floor is becoming increasingly recognised as a cause of incontinence.

Ageing of elastic and collagen connective tissue surrounding the urethra may partly explain why urethral closing pressure reduces with increasing age. In post-menopausal women the hormonal changes responsible for the changes of atrophic vaginitis may also produce epithelial changes in the urethra and trigone as well as changes in elastic connective tissue in the urethral wall. In men the major anatomical change with age is benign prostatic enlargement.

History of Urinary Incontinence

The history taken from any elderly patient should include specific questions about incontinence of both urine and faeces. It is useful to preface questions with a statement to the effect that problems with control of bowels and "waterworks" are common in older people and it is important to find out about them because treatment is generally successful in helping with the problems. Such a positive approach indicates to the patient that the questioner takes the problem seriously and wants to help with it.

The time course of urinary incontinence may give valuable information. Recent onset of incontinence with falls or confusion may indicate the presence of an underlying neurological illness. The incontinence may represent the summation of age-related changes in bladder control and a new neurological disorder. The patient who first becomes incontinent at the time of a myocardial infarction may cross the threshold of incontinence as a result of reduction in cerebral blood flow involving the micturition centre, as a result of enforced bed rest (the patient being "imprisoned" and hence unable to get to the toilet), or because a diuretic results at some time during the day in a rate of urine production greater than can be coped with by the patient's unstable bladder, which then contracts uncontrollably. Thus it is important to assess the whole range of factors likely to be relevant and catheterisation must not be allowed to become the long-term solution to incontinence. If possible it should be avoided altogether.

The time of day when incontinence occurs may indicate the cause or potential management strategy. Nocturnal incontinence in isolation is usually due to an unstable bladder. Incontinence a few hours after administration of diuretic is easily explained. One must beware of the patient who is incontinent during the day without obvious physical cause but is completely continent at night – the incontinence may be a manipulative gesture or a "dirty protest" at an unaccept-able life situation; such patients may become continent as soon as they are admitted to hospital – a useful marker in diagnosis and management.

The severity of the incontinence may also give clues to its cause. Patients with unstable bladder are intermittently incontinent, whereas those with retention with overflow leak urine continously.

It is important to ask the patient about factors which seem to precipitate episodes of incontinence. Coughing, sneezing, laughing and changes in posture may lead to incontinence in individuals with true stress incontinence or with the so-called "pseudo stress incontinence" found in some patients with unstable bladders: these conditions will be discussed in more detail later, but if the patient indicates that the precipitant leads to loss of only a small amount of urine ("less than an eggcupful") then the likely diagnosis is true stress inconti-nence, whereas loss of larger volumes of urine suggests the presence of an unstable bladder.

The incontinent patient should be asked about bowel function. One of the most easily treated causes of urinary incontinence is severe constipation with faecal impaction leading to retention with overflow. The patient may not admit or complain of constipation, particularly if she is demented. She may have been referred with urinary and faecal incontinence of recent onset and if the latter is incontinence of very loose or liquid faeces then the cause of the double incontinence is often faecal impaction.

Symptoms of urinary tract disease are common in elderly females and do not necessarily relate to underlying pathology. The presence of dysuria (which in a younger person would be taken as evidence of urinary tract infection) is less significant in the elderly and is found in many women in whom the urine is sterile: loin or suprapubic pain of recent onset is more suggestive of acute infection.

General features of the patient's condition, especially mobility, mental state and ease of getting to the toilet are all–important in the assessment of the incontinent patient. Many incontinent patients tend to drink less, especially in the evening, on the assumption that a lower fluid intake will produce less urine and hence reduce the tendency to incontinence: in fact, although the urine volume is reduced, the urine is more concentrated and this may increase the incontinence. Advice to drink more may result in a reduction or even cessation of incontinence, much to the surprise and delight of the patient.

Examination and Investigation

As with all problems in the elderly a full physical examination is required. Much of this has been dealt with in Chapter 1 and here only points particularly pertinent to the patient who is incontinent of urine will be covered.

All incontinent patients should be examined rectally to detect faecal impac-tion and, in men, prostatic enlargement or malignancy. Women should be examined for stress or pseudo stress incontinence by observing the external urethral meatus while the patient coughs or strains downwards. This may be achieved with the patient recumbent, but failure to demonstrate urethral leakage of urine in this position indicates the need to repeat the examination with the patient standing. In true stress incontinence a short sharp spurt of urine is lost through the urethra during the cough. In pseudo stress incontinence, where the cause is a myelopathy, the initial rise in intra-abdominal pressure triggers a detrusor contraction resulting in a prolonged stream of urine which gradually subsides. Most patients will distinguish between these alternative forms of stress incontinence by reporting, in the former, the voiding of only small quantities of urine, whereas in the latter case the patient will describe "a flood".

Culture of the urine should be undertaken in all incontinent patients. It is unusual for infection alone to be responsible for incontinence in the elderly but, if the patient has underlying bladder instability, infection may cause bladder irritation sufficient to render the patient incontinent.

Although a distended bladder may be detected by palpation, it is often missed in obese patients. Measurement of residual urine by catheterisation after micturition should resolve the question but in the patient with dribbling or overflow incontinence, a plain abdominal X-ray examination will demonstrate bladder distension and will also show whether the patient has "high" impaction of faeces: in this condition rectal examination is normal but X-ray examination shows heavy faecal loading higher in the descending and sigmoid colon.

Charting of incontinence through the day together with regular two hourly toiletting is essential. Using this method for a number of days not only highlights problem times during the day but also establishes whether regular toiletting will result in the patient staying dry.

The cause of incontinence can be diagnosed in most patients by a careful history and examination coupled with the simple investigations so far described. Pressure studies should be used selectively and invasive investigation of demented patients in whom the incontinence is likely to be due to the pathological process underlying the dementia is inappropriate and distressing to the patient. In such patients therapeutic trials of drugs and of simple techniques to control the incontinence may be much more satisfactory. Cystoscopy and intravenous urography may be required in the diagnosis of urinary tract pathology and occasionally in women the cytology of the vaginal epithelium may provide information about the endocrine status of the female genital tract and help to establish whether senile vaginitis is at least partly responsible for the incontinence.

The Causes of Urinary Incontinence

A unitary diagnostic approach to urinary incontinence in the elderly is inappropriate because patients commonly have several contributing factors; for example, the patient may have a paraparesis but may require treatment directed towards her stress incontinence, senile vaginitis and urinary tract infection.

The causes of urinary incontinence in the elderly can be separated into two groups – mechanical causes and neurological causes. Conditions such as prolapse, prostatism and atrophic vaginitis are common but are not the subject of this book. Neurological causes of incontinence may be classified as frontal lobe incontinence, upper spinal cord lesions and cauda equina or lumbo-sacral plexus lesions.

Frontal Lobe Incontinence

Patients with lesions affecting the parasagittal cerebral cortex in the frontal lobe in the region of the anterior cingulate gyri develop a characteristic disorder of continence. There is no warning of the need to empty the bladder and the patient is surprised but usually indifferent to the sudden involuntary emptying of the bladder. The early symptoms of this type of incontinence may mimic spinal lesions with urgency and precipitancy of micturition but the distinction can usually be made by the lack of any warning of impending incontinence in the frontal type, and the lack of any sense of embarrassment that these patients show. Parasagittal frontal tumour, especially meningioma, may present in this way. Frontal lobe incontinence is also a cardinal sign of normal pressure hydrocephalus.

Where the condition has developed as the result of stroke or where there is a progressive dementing disorder or inoperable tumour, treatment is rarely successful. Some patients can be helped at least temporarily by training them to empty their bladder two or three hourly "by the clock". Anticholinergic drugs seldom have a place in the treatment of this form of incontinence.

Upper Spinal Lesions

Upper spinal lesions, whether compressive, vascular or degenerative, will lead to an evolution of urinary symptoms culminating in incontinence and dependent on the severity of the disorder. Initially the patient may become aware only of slight hesitancy of initiation of micturition. Later urgency, frequency and finally precipitancy with incontinence or pseudo stress incontinence will develop. These symptoms may easily be confused with symptoms of prostatism or stress incontinence. Examination must, therefore, always be directed towards assessing for the presence of mechanical abnormalities associated with the symptoms (prostatic hypertrophy in the male, prolapse in the female), and to eliciting neurological signs of pyramidal deficit (spastic weakness of the lower limbs with extensor plantar responses) which normally accompany this form of incontinence.

Spinal cord lesions causing bladder disturbance require careful clinical assessment and investigation. But symptomatic treatment of the incontinence may be the only therapeutic option that is available.

For many patients in the early stages of the condition toiletting may be all that is required, together with advice about drinking adequate amounts of liquid. It may be necessary to supplement day-time toiletting with toiletting at night with the help of an appropriately timed alarm clock. Patients who continue to be incontinent at night may require either anticholinergic medication to reduce spontaneous bladder contractions or the provision of incontinence devices or garments.

Anticholinergic Agents. A number of these have been used including imipramine, propantheline, dicyclomine, oxybutynin, terodiline and orphenadrine hydrochloride. If the drug is taken during the day-time, detrusor activity is reduced with corresponding reduction in urgency and frequency. If taken in the late evening enuresis or nocturia may be avoidable.

These drugs all share the disadvantage that they may induce or exacerbate symptoms of confusion often accompanied by hallucinations. In patients with mental impairment their use is therefore limited. Dry mouth, dysphagia and blurring of vision are other occasional side effects. Glaucoma is a contra-indication to the use of these drugs.

Cauda Equina and Lumbo-sacral Plexus Lesions
Compressive lesions of the lowermost segments of the spinal cord, or cauda equina, are seen in elderly patients with central prolapsed disc, epidural spinal deposits from malignant disease, Paget's disease or destructive processes affecting the lumbar vertebrae (e.g., myeloma) or malignant meningitis. Those conditions, in which the bony skeleton or intervertebral discs or joints are affected, are usually painful, whereas epidural deposits and malignant meningitis may be painless.

The neurological signs are those of lumbo-sacral root lesion(s) with lower motor neurone weakness and areflexia in the appropriate segments associated with dermatome sensory loss. Bladder dysfunction is typically that of loss of bladder sensation with flaccid distension of the bladder and overflow incontinence. Urethral sensation during micturition will be lost if sacral segments S2, 3, 4 are involved.

Atonic neurogenic bladder is occasionally seen in elderly patients due to destruction of sensory fibres in diabetic neuropathy, autonomic neuropathies or, classically, in tabes dorsalis in which posterior nerve roots are destroyed. Some power to micturate voluntarily remains, but the patient is so unaware of bladder filling that bladder distension occurs to the point at which retention with overflow develops. This cause of incontinence is treated by training the patient to empty the bladder using suprapubic pressure and regular two or three hourly voiding "by the clock".

Faecal Incontinence

Faecal incontinence is often found in association with urinary incontinence. The relationship between the two may occur when faecal impaction causes retention with overflow of both urine and faeces; urinary and faecal incontinence also coexist in demented patients, the rectum behaving in a similar fashion to the unstable bladder. In demented patients urinary incontinence almost invariably precedes faecal incontinence. Faecal incontinence occuring de novo in the absence of urinary incontinence is an indicator of underlying bowel pathology.

Normal Control of Defaecation

As with the bladder, the spinal reflexes which control rectal activity are subject to inhibitory control from higher levels in the CNS including the cerebrum. The reflex arcs responsible for rectal control are situated in S3 and 4. The ano-rectal region is composed of two distinct parts, the "visceral" part which is the termination of smooth muscle layers in the gut and which is autonomically innervated via plexuses in the gut wall, and an outer "somatic" striated muscle component. The most important part of the latter is the puborectalis muscle, which acts as a sling anchoring the rectum to the pubis and thus maintains the ano-rectal junction at a right angle; this creates a flap valve over the anal canal, which is largely responsible for the maintenance of faecal continence. The somatic component also includes the external anal sphincter and the other muscles of the pelvic floor.

Little is known about specific changes due to ageing which affect the ano-rectal region. Higher control of defaecation seems to be subject to similar problems in old age to the higher control of micturition. Causes of faecal incontinence are summarised in Table 7.1.

Table 7.1. Causes of faecal incontinence

1. *Abnormal intestinal activity* or damage to pelvic floor
   Diarrhoea   Inflammatory bowel disease
                                Tumour
   Faecal impaction
   Trauma, Surgery

2. *Loss of control of anal sphincter*
a) Cerebral
      Dementia
      Frontal lesions   Parasagittal tumour
                                Stroke
                                Binswanger's encephalopathy
b) Spinal
      Compressive spinal cord lesions
         Extradural metastases
         Bone lesions
            Pagets disease
            Metastases
            Tuberculosis
            Osteomyelitis
         Canal stenosis
         Cervical spondylosis
c) Lumbo-sacral plexopathy
      Pelvic carcinoma or lymphoma
      Post *Herpes zoster*
      Atonia of levator ani

3. *Behavioural causes*
   "Dirty protest"

History of Faecal Incontinence

The length of time that a patient had been incontinent gives some indication whether the incontinence is a new and acute problem, perhaps associated with a diarrhoeal illness, or a chronic condition perhaps due to loss of higher control or to local bowel pathology. If the incontinence has been present for many years without other obvious problems it may, as described below, be due to weakness of the pelvic floor.

A history of recent constipation suggests that faecal impaction may have occurred either as a result of other illness (for example a chest infection) perhaps resulting in immobility, or because of a local lesion in the bowel causing obstruction and consequent overflow of liquid faeces.

In the presence of other neurological signs of paraparesis, faecal incontinence may indicate a compressive lesion of the spinal cord.

The frequency of faecal incontinence and the consistency of the stools may give some indication of the underlying cause. Constant soiling, particularly of very loose stool, is consistent with faecal impaction and overflow. Irregular incontinence of formed stool, especially after meals or hot drinks suggests loss of higher control and an "unstable rectum".

Neurological disorders leading to this form of faecal incontinence may be cerebral spinal or lumbo-sacral. Spinal lesions will characteristically show the signs of pyramidal weakness in the legs and there is usually impairment of bladder and rectal sensation. In lumbo-sacral plexus lesions (e.g. due to pelvic carcinoma) the sensory symptoms and signs predominate with anaesthesia in the sacral dermatomes and a patulous atonic external anal sphincter.

As mentioned above, coexisting or preceding urinary incontinence is an important feature in both faecal impaction, for whatever cause, and in demented patients; in the latter the dual incontinence usually reflecting loss of higher control.

A history of diabetes may indicate that the patient has diarrhoea due to impairment of autonomic control of the bowel from diabetic neuropathy. The characteristic pattern is nocturnal diarrhoea or incontinence. Only rarely is there associated autonomic neuropathic disturbance of the bladder.

Poor fluid intake can lead to constipation, as can poor intake of food. Excessive alcohol consumption is also important since many elderly people who drink to excess may suffer with diarrhoea and incontinence of faeces.

Examination

Abdominal palpation may indicate faecal masses in the colon or other masses due to intra-abdominal pathology. Rectal examination will reveal the degree of anal tone, whether the rectum is empty or not, and the consistency of the stool. In severe retention of faeces the anus may be gaping due to the faecal mass simulating denervation of the anal sphincter. Tumours and strictures may be palpable rectally. Perianal sensation must always be tested.

Conclusion

Problems associated with loss of control of elimination are amongst the most sensitive and distressing found in medical practice. They are consistently hidden by patients and unsought by doctors, many of whom regard them as "uninteresting" compared to conditions which can be investigated and treated using more sophisticated techniques. For the patient whose problem is identified and properly managed, however, the benefit is inestimable. For the doctor, incontinence presents an opportunity to exercise clinical skills of the very highest order and a considerable diagnostic and therapeutic challenge spanning a wide range of medical knowledge and specialties.

8 Parkinsonism and Abnormal Movement Disorders

The descriptive word "Parkinsonism" covers a constellation of disorders that are age-related and present a series of common problems in clinical practice. In the normal elderly person, increased flexion of the trunk and a shortening of the pace in walking are commonly observed. These physical signs are features of parkinsonism and there is frequently difficulty in distinguishing between age-related changes and parkinsonism, especially in the very old. Similarly slowness of movement and mentation (retardation/bradyphrenia) are features of both depressive illness and parkinsonism; and depressive symptoms are so common in Parkinson's disease as to be regarded by some as a normal feature of that condition. The diagnosis of parkinsonism is therefore difficult. It is even more difficult clinically to identify within this group of akinetic-rigid syndromes those patients who have idiopathic parkinsonism or Parkinson's disease. Post-mortem analysis reveals that approximately 25% of the brains from patients diagnosed as Parkinson's disease in life show neuropathological changes incompatible with that diagnosis.

There are a multiplicity of presenting symptoms of the akinetic-rigid syndrome which we call parkinsonism. There have already been mentioned changes in posture and gait, and depressive symptoms and their lack of specificity have been emphasised. Similarly symptoms of slowness, tiredness, "weakness", balance disturbance, stiffness, difficulty in rising from a low chair, pain in the neck, back or shoulder, awkwardness getting into a car or bath, speech disturbance, clumsiness and loss of dexterity are all non-specific symptoms but are also the usual presenting symptoms of parkinsonism. Tremor, as a symptom, is non-specific but too often it is seized upon by patient and physician alike and regarded as a diagnostic feature of parkinsonism. Tremor, as a sign on examination, if it fulfils the clinical criteria for parkinsonian tremor, is indeed a diagnostic feature. But it is often difficult to distinguish between parkinsonian tremor and benign essential tremor in the elderly and, incidentally, the effect of drug treatment is an unreliable way of making this distinction.

There are two stages in the diagnosis. It is first necessary to establish that the patient's symptoms (however non-specific or even apparently irrelevant) are associated with the classical clinical features of parkinsonism – rigidity, bradykinesia, and possibly tremor. (Tremor is not essential for the diagnosis, indeed it is frequently entirely absent in classical Parkinson's disease.) Second, it is necessary to decide which of the disorders grouped within the parkinsonian syndrome or "parkinsonism" accounts for the disability in the patient. At this second stage an aetiological diagnosis may be possible – for example, drug-induced parkinsonism or multi-infarct cerebral degeneration.

These two stages of diagnosis should be consciously gone through in order to reach a proper assessment of prognosis and management. Spot diagnosis seems impressive but, unless it is backed up with careful examination, it can lead to wrong diagnosis and incorrect treatment. It also leads to incorrect advice for patient and family, particularly with regard to therapeutic expectations and prognosis.

With the advent of effective medical treatment for Parkinson's disease the condition has become over-diagnosed. Doctors and patients alike want to diagnose Parkinson's disease because it holds much less fear and therapeutic nihilism than closely related disorders such as Alzheimer's disease or even old age. But to make an incorrect diagnosis of Parkinson's disease leads to an inaccurate prognosis and to faulty management which, at best, may involve unnecessary therapy and, at worst, may expose the patient to dangerous or unpleasant side effects. Although the condition is overdiagnosed it is none-the-less common.

The prevalence of parkinsonism in general and Parkinson's disease in particular rises with increasing age. Thus a prevalence of about 0.1% below the age of 60 years rises to a prevalence of about 1% in those aged over 70 years, and may reach an incidence as high as 2.5% or more in those aged 85 years and over. With modern treatment patients with Parkinson's disease are surviving longer so that the excess mortality from this condition (compared with age and sex-matched control patients) is now about 1.5 in the over 65 year-old-group compared with 3.0 before the advent of levodopa.

Parkinsonism is largely a disease of the elderly. Nearly 60% of sufferers are aged 70 years or over. While the diagnosis must always be borne in mind, care must therefore be exercised to reach a correct diagnosis in every case.

Assessment of severity of the disease is always essential, especially in the elderly where it dictates the need for social and domestic support services. It is not sufficient to label the condition "parkinsonism" and "try the effect" of the dopamine agonists and other drugs recommended for Parkinson's disease. Decisions about the type of medication to be used, dosage and drug combinations; decisions about occupational, speech and physiotherapy; and decisions about domestic environment and support services all depend on the assessment of severity of the disease, rate of progression and the particular circumstances and personality of the individual.

The Presenting Symptoms and Signs of Parkinsonism

It is commonplace for patients or their spouses to attribute the early symptoms of parkinsonism to old age. It is accepted that people "slow up" as they get older, so the slowness of voluntary movement and the mental lethargy that goes with it are easily blamed on *anno domini* rather than perceived as part of a pathological process.

The diagnosis is often made by an astute doctor seeing the patient for some unrelated reason and noting the classical features of parkinsonism almost in passing. The closer you are to the patient the less obvious these features may be. Like hypothyroidism the diagnosis of parkinsonism may escape the general practitioner who sees the patient frequently, but be obvious to the Accident and Emergency surgeon seeing the patient for the first time – but perhaps for an injury that could have been avoided if the parkinsonism had been considered; doubt often persists even after a careful examination of the patient. Parkinson's disease and the related disorders remain a clinical diagnosis where confirmation of the diagnosis is seldom available during life. What, then, are the features on which a diagnosis of parkinsonism is made?

Where tremor is the presenting symptom, the possible diagnosis will be obvious and only requires confirmation. But tremor is less common in the elderly with parkinsonism than it is in the younger patient and presenting symptoms of weakness or fatiguability are probably the most frequently seen. The arm is first noticed to have lost fine movement so that the patient notices a difficulty with writing or sewing if the dominant hand is affected first or with dressing or playing the piano if the left hand is first affected. The upper limb tends to be affected before the lower limb when the complaint may be difficulty in lifting the foot up with a tendency to trip over the edge of a carpet. Disturbance of balance combined with "weakness" of a leg may lead to the patient presenting with falls or difficulty getting in to a car.

Case 8.1
A 68-year-old retired Army officer first became aware of significant symptoms when he slipped into a shallow ditch while out shooting and found himself unable to scramble up the bank. Friends had already noticed a slowing up but had attributed it to old age.

When the patient is questioned an inability to hurry is often admitted. And a specific difficulty in turning over in bed is remarkably characteristic of the disorder.

True weakness is absent on examination in Parkinson's disease – that is, there is no loss of power, such as would prevent the patient lifting or carrying a heavy load. The complaint of fatiguability may suggest myasthenia but on examination although voluntary movements, particularly repetitive movements such as polishing furniture or tapping, decline in rate and range, the increasing weakness on sustained effort seen in myasthenia gravis is absent in parkinsonism. And strength does not recover rapidly with rest in Parkinson's disease as it does in myasthenia.

The parkinsonian patient enters the consulting room typically with a posture of slight flexion of the neck and a round shouldered stance which is reminiscent of old age. The gait tends to be abnormal with the weight thrown slightly too far forward and the length of pace reduced. These signs may suggest parkinsonism before the patient has mentioned a symptom. The facies often gives the appearance of being younger than the chronological age of the patient. The skin may be less wrinkled than would be expected and slightly seborrhoeic. There is usually reduced blinking and reduced play of facial expression especially in the upper half of the face, associated with a generalised reduction of associated movements. Most patients visiting a doctor will exhibit some nervousness but the parkinsonian does not move his head and trunk but sits quietly and relatively immobile. There are no nervous mannerisms of the hands or shuffling of the feet.

These signs of hypokinesia are more significant in diagnosis than those elicited in examination. But slowness of fine movements of the fingers or tapping movements at the wrist will usually bring out the features of bradykinesia and confirm the diagnosis. The handwriting will be small and tends to decrease in size and legibility the longer it is continued. Speech may be soft, slow and monotonous with a tendency to stutter.

Rigidity is the other cardinal sign of parkinsonism but is asymptomatic. However, it is probable that the pain of Parkinson's disease is related to the rigidity of the muscles. Certainly pain is a common symptom in parkinsonism, especially before treatment is initiated. It is felt in the neck, shoulder and back and will mimic other musculo-skeletal disorders of old age – osteoarthritis or polymyalgia.

The parkinsonian disorders of gait are among the most important in elderly patients with this condition. Even early in the disease it is common to find a difficulty in turning, and a slight hesitancy when starting to walk. Some patients find that their pace progressively shortens especially when walking indoors and negotiating the obstructions of furniture. "Freezing" episodes may lead to falling with the patient unable to put his hands out to save himself. Occasionally the progressively shortening step combined with the tendency to lean forward will lead to the characteristic "propensity . . . to pass from walking to a running pace" (James Parkinson 1817).

In the elderly, bladder symptoms, incontinence, constipation and symptoms of memory failure, thought block or even frank dementia are common. They are mentioned here because with eye signs, blood pressure problems, drug history, history of trauma, and features of arteriosclerosis they may indicate the specific type of parkinsonism from which the patient is suffering.

The Examination of the Patient with Parkinsonism

The Tremor

In Parkinson's disease there is typically a 4–6 Hz resting tremor of the upper limb, which disappears with sustained posture or voluntary movement. It is usually asymmetrical and under partial voluntary control. It is made worse by nervousness. It is much less common in Parkinson's disease presenting in old age than in younger patients.

Parkinsonian tremor needs to be distinguished chiefly from essential tremor which is more rapid (8–12 hz), disappears on full relaxation and tends to be maximal on sustained posture. Essential tremor is usually relieved temporarily by alcohol. It may be inherited as an autosomal dominant but has none of the associated akinetic-rigid features of parkinsonism. However essential tremor is common in old age and may co-exist with parkinsonism.

Hypokinesia

Two closely related phenomena are characteristic of parkinsonism.

1. A slowness of willed movement or bradykinesia
2. An inability to initiate a willed movement or the tendency for that willed movement to become arrested involuntarily – akinesia

While bradykinesia tends, therefore, to affect all forms of voluntary movement in the activities of daily living, akinesia tends to affect those activities which require sustained or repetitive movement such as walking, writing, speech or polishing/brushing teeth–type movements.

The phenomenon of hypokinesia is associated with a paucity or loss of associated movements – facial expression, arm swing, and "body language".

In the elderly patient hypokinesia tends to be symmetrical and to affect the trunk and mid-line musculature. Thus symptoms of slowness of movement in rising from a chair, turning over in bed, turning the head and slowness and softness of speech predominate over unilateral loss of dexterity often seen in the younger patient.

Rigidity

"Rigidity" is the sense of resistance felt by the examiner when a limb of the patient is passively moved. Classically this resistance is either constant throughout the range of movement or has the regularly variable quality aptly called "cogwheel". Rigidity generally is first noticeable in the shoulder or elbow and only later in wrist, fingers or lower limb. Where rigidity is minimal it will be exacerbated by subjecting the patient to stress such as asking him to perform mental arithmetic or by instructing him to carry out manipulations with the contralateral limb.

Like hypokinesia, rigidity has a greater tendency to affect both arms in the elderly compared with the early onset case where rigidity may affect one arm only. Similarly rigidity of the neck muscles is seen in the senile case where it is uncommon in younger patients.

Other Signs in Parkinsonism

Tremor, hypokinesia and rigidity are the diagnostic "core" signs of parkinsonism. The many other signs seen in this group of disorders tend to be seen with greater or less frequency or severity in different types of the disorder. At this stage, therefore, the classification of the disease in Table 8.1 needs to be borne in mind. Thus gait disturbances are especially important in senile parkinsonism, and multi-infarct disease. Cognitive changes are also common in these forms of the condition, but are even more prominent in Alzheimer's disease, cortico-basal degeneration and Steele–Richardson syndrome, but may occur in multi-infarct parkinsonism and post-encephalitic disease. Nigro-striatal degeneration is a diagnosis that can normally only be made on pathological grounds post-mortem.

Disorders of Gait

Characteristically the parkinsonian starts with a posture flexed at all joints (the so-called "simian" posture) and has difficulty in starting to walk. She may describe this difficulty as a feeling of the "feet stuck to the floor". In trying to start walking, she may topple forward and either fall or "chase her centre of gravity" with rapid, small paces. The gait is characterised by small steps and reduced arm swing. Turning requires multiple small movements of the feet. There is a tendency for walking to come to an involuntary halt, especially at the threshold of a door or minor obstruction, e.g., furniture. Conversely and paradoxically patients with parkinsonism often find it easier to walk upstairs where the length of their pace is determined by the tread.

Table 8.1. Classification of disorders in the elderly leading to an akinetic-rigid state ("parkinsonism")

Primary idiopathic parkinsonism
 Parkinson's disease
 Senile parkinsonism or diffuse Lewy body disease
 Striato-nigral degeneration

Degenerative disorders with parkinsonism
 Multi-system atrophy (incl. Shy–Drager and olivo-ponto-cerebellar degeneration)
 Steele–Richardson–Olszewski syndrome (progressive supranuclear palsy)
 Alzheimer's disease
 Cortico-basal degeneration

Parkinsonism of known aetiology
 Multi-infarct disease (arteriosclerotic parkinsonism)
 Drugs – phenothiazines, butyrophenones, tetrabenazine, MPTP
 Traumatic (boxers) encephalopathy
 Postencephalitic parkinsonism
 Manganese poisoning

Disorders of Higher Mental Function

In some patients depression is clearly reactive and secondary to the physical disability. But in the majority the depression of Parkinson's disease is endogenous in type. It is so common as to be a usual feature in the primary idiopathic parkinsonisms.

Akathisia is a behavioural disorder associated with the drug-induced disorder and the primary and post-encephalitic parkinsonisms. It is characterised by a compulsive restlessness. In the day-time the patient feels compelled to get out of the chair and walk round the room. As soon as she is on her feet the symptom declines only to return when she sits down. At night the patient may lie awake tortured by akathisia because she is unable to turn over or get out of bed. Eventually she will wake her spouse to help her out of bed where an unnecessary visit to the toilet is made the excuse.

"Thought block" (where in mid-conversation the parkinsonian suddenly loses the thread of what he is saying) and bradyphrenia or slowness of mental activity are both characteristic symptoms of primary parkinsonism. Cognitive deterioration with memory failure, apathy, and profound slowness of mentation is a common feature in senile parkinsonism of the diffuse cortical Lewy-body type, as well as Alzheimer's disease, Steele–Richardson syndrome and multi-infarct disease. In geriatric practice, where diffuse cortical Lewy-body disease is common, dementia developing early in the disease and progressing inexorably causes some of the most difficult problems of management (see below).

Autonomic Function

Seborrhoea is a common feature of Parkinson's disease and post-encephalitic parkinsonism. Other disturbances of autonomic function – postural hypotension, bladder disturbance and constipation – are characteristic of the multi-system atrophies, where they may be the presenting symptoms, but they are also an important group of symptoms in senile parkinsonism.

Postural hypotension is an important cause of fainting and falling. It also may lead to impaired cerebral perfusion with forgetfulness and mild confusion, unsteadiness and symptoms of weakness and faintness. In the elderly, blood pressure lying and standing should be checked regularly. The dopamine agonists share a tendency to exacerbate postural hypotension thereby limiting their usefulness in some cases.

Bladder disturbance in parkinsonism usually consists of symptoms of frequency and urgency but occasionally hesitancy and retention of urine predominate. In the former group detrusor hyperreflexia appears to be the pathophysiological basis; whereas in cases of hesitancy and retention sphincter bradykinesia with or without partial bladder de-afferentation (in multi-system atrophy) probably accounts for the symptoms.

Constipation is commonplace in the elderly patient suffering from any locomotor disorder. It is particularly common in parkinsonism, where autonomic changes are often exacerbated by anticholinergic medication. Constipation should be separately assessed in patients with parkinsonism and it should be treated independently of the main treatment plan for the parkinsonian signs.

Hypersalivation with dribbling is not strictly an autonomic disturbance but is common as a feature of parkinsonism. It is due to reduced involuntary swallowing which, when associated with a flexed posture, means that accumulating saliva dribbles from the front of the mouth.

Eye Signs

In progressive supranuclear palsy (Steele–Richardson syndrome) a gaze palsy, affecting vertical eye movements particularly, is an early and prominent feature. In Parkinson's disease convergence of the eyes is often impaired and in post-encephalitic parkinsonism a variety of eye movement disorders may be seen of which the most characteristic is the oculo-gyric crisis. In senile parkinsonism impairment of conjugate upward gaze and convergence is common but whether this feature is independent of the condition and merely age-related is uncertain.

The eye signs of parkinsonism are not amenable to drug treatment.

Assessment

The examination of the patient should allow a clinical diagnosis as to the cause of the parkinsonism (Table 8.1). This is important because it determines treatment and prognosis. The primary signs of parkinsonism should be assessed for severity by using a simple rating scale which will allow the progress of the disease to be followed over time. Thus rigidity, tremor and bradykinesia may be separately assessed for right and left side, with ratings as follows: 0, normal; 1, mild; 2, moderate; 3, severe degrees of abnormality. The response of the patient to treatment can also be annotated by this means. In the elderly it is particularly important also to assess quantitatively gait disturbance and dementia. The common levodopa complications of "on-off" attacks and dyskinesia are difficult to measure in terms of severity but should also be included in any outpatient assessment.

Course

The primary parkinsonisms and the degenerative disorders associated with parkinsonism follow a progressive course and this is not known to be influenced by any of the treatments currently available. The rate of deterioration tends to be constant in the individual case without acceleration or plateau of disability.

In the elderly two forms of parkinsonism predominate, Parkinson's disease and senile parkinsonism of the diffuse Lewy-body type – and the remainder of this chapter will concentrate on these.

Parkinson's Disease and Senile Parkinsonism

Parkinson's disease tends to present before the age of 65 years. There is a slight male predominance and the disease usually progresses slowly. Senile parkinsonism usually develops after the age of 70 years, the sex incidence is equal and the disease progresses more rapidly, with increasing disability and dependency.

Response to dopamine agonists is usually excellent in Parkinson's disease, but the early relief of symptoms is followed within a few years by the development of fluctuations in response, wearing-off effects and dyskinesia in the majority. The patient with senile parkinsonism, however, responds less well to dopamine agonists with only partial relief of symptoms. Dose levels in senile parkinsonism are often restricted by symptoms of confusion or hypotension but dyskinesia and response fluctuations are rare and not severe. Dementia is a characteristic feature of senile parkinsonism. It may precede the parkinsonian signs or it may not develop until the parkinsonism has been established for several years. However, the development of dementia in senile parkinsonism has a profound effect on management and prognosis so that life expectancy in this form of the disease is less than two years from the development of dementia.

Alzheimer's disease may co-exist with Parkinson's disease, usually developing after Parkinson's disease has been present for a few years. Clinically the two disorders may have a different tempo of progression but, in practice, this combination may be difficult or impossible to distinguish from senile parkinsonism.

In the management of the elderly patient with parkinsonism of the idiopathic type it is important to make a distinction between senile and idiopathic (classical) Parkinson's disease. The pathological differences can only be made by histological examination, when idiopathic Parkinson's disease shows the characteristic intra-neuronal Lewy body inclusions restricted to the brainstem and basal nuclei and affecting the substantia nigra in particular, whereas in senile parkinsonism Lewy bodies are found diffusely through the brain, but they affect the cerebral cortical neurones as well as those of the substantia nigra.

The differential clinical features are perhaps best exemplified by two case histories.

Case 8.2
Now aged 79 years, this patient presented with tremor and slight unilateral hypokinesia 19 years ago when she was aged 60 years. Treatment with levodopa was started 4 years later with immediate dramatic response. However, within

2 years she had developed intermittent facial and limb dyskinesias which have persisted and worsened ever since.

She now has severe dyskinetic and dystonic side effects from her levodopa, but in spite of these runs a large house (she was widowed a year ago) and looks after the garden. She is entirely independent and her mental state is normal. For a total of about an hour every day she suffers from unpredictable "off"attacks, each lasting 10–20 minutes.

Case 8.3
Also 79 years of age, this female first developed mild generalised hypokinesia and rigidity 3 years ago. The signs were those of classical hypokinetic parkinsonism without tremor. She was not demented and was looking after an elderly, partially disabled husband.

Response to levodopa treatment was moderate with improvement in speed of walking, dressing and preparing food. The parkinsonian symptoms progressed over 18 months, in spite of rising medication. She then began to become forgetful and apathetic. Within 12 months she was frankly demented and had to be admitted for continuing nursing care with moderately severe physical features of parkinsonism.

Management

The distinction between Parkinson's disease and senile parkinsonism with diffuse Lewy body formation may be difficult or impossible clinically until features of dementia are evident. And at the time of diagnosis this is unusual. The clinical features listed in Table 8.2 may allow a working diagnosis which will provide a guide to management. Before a decision is made as to the regime of treatment to recommend an assessment of severity should be made. Four

Table 8.2. A comparison of the features of idiopathic with senile parkinsonism

	Parkinson's disease	Senile parkinsonism
Pathology	Lewy-body formation restricted to the brainstem and basal nuclei	Diffuse Lewy body formation in brainstem, basal nuclei and cortex
Age of onset (years)	< 65	> 70
Sex ratio	M > F	M = F
Progression	Slow	Moderate or rapid
Tremor	Common	Uncommon
Rigidity and bradykinesia	Asymmetrical	Symmetrical
Posture and balance	Affected late	Affected early and progressive
Response to therapy	Good	Moderate to poor
On-Off fluctuations and dyskinesias	Common within 5 yr	Rare, mild and late
Dementia	Rare	Common

broad categories of severity are helpful:

1. *Mild.* The patient has symptoms of parkinsonism but no disability
2. *Moderate.* The patient has disability from parkinsonism but remains independent in activities of daily living
3. *Severe.* The patient is so severely afflicted as to be dependent on others for activities of daily living
4. *Terminal.* Specific therapy cannot influence the patient's condition to any significant extent

Patients with Parkinson's disease may not require treatment at all when they present with disease at the "mild" stage, but they should remain under regular outpatient review to assess the rate of deterioration of their condition. If treatment is desirable because the symptoms are distressing or limiting, an anticholinergic drug and/or amantadine should be advised. When the disease progresses to the "moderate" stage it is necessary to introduce a dopamine agonist – either levodopa with decarboxylase inhibitor (Madopar or Sinemet) or bromocriptine. Levodopa is better tolerated than bromocriptine; but bromocriptine when used de novo (prior to the patient being treated with levodopa) does not seem to cause the fluctuations of response or dyskinesia that are so troublesome with levodopa. Whichever drug is used, it should be introduced in minimal dosage and taken after meals, and the doses should be increased slowly until the disabling symptoms are relieved. Anticholinergics should probably be continued at the "moderate" and at the "severe" stage unless side effects develop. When the patient is suffering from severe symptoms of the disease maximum tolerated dose of levodopa with or without bromocriptine and anticholinergics should be used. At this stage the major problem in Parkinson's disease is usually fluctuations of response, where the patient quite abruptly becomes hypokinetic and rigid and loses all the effect of their treatment for a period of 10–60 minutes. These "on-off" fluctuations may be impossible to avoid completely, but frequent small doses of levodopa may provide some relief and combined treatment with levodopa and bromocriptine may also mitigate this problem. It is often useful to chart motor fluctuations through the day in order to judge the optimum timing of levodopa dosage. The drug treatment of idiopathic parkinsonism is summarised in Table 8.3.

Diffuse Lewy body disease or senile parkinsonism should be treated differently from idiopathic parkinsonism. The patient is usually elderly and the risk of levodopa fluctuations and dyskinesias is less, but these patients tend to develop confusional states with anticholinergics and bromocriptine. They should therefore be treated with levodopa with decarboxylase inhibitor from the outset and the dose should be increased according to the progression of the disease.

Dyskinesias which are common in the later stages of the dopa-treated disease are difficult to control. They are not painful but are socially conspicuous and may exhaust the patient. They can only be relieved by reducing the dose of levodopa and this inevitably leads to a return of parkinsonism.

Selegiline is a monoamine oxidase B inhibitor and probably acts by slowing the breakdown of dopamine and its action is, therefore, slightly to increase and

Table 8.3. The drug treatment of idiopathic parkinsonism

	Mild	Moderate	Severe	Terminal
Parkinson's disease	Nil or Benzhexol Amantadine	Benzhexol and levodopa (+DCI) or Bromocriptine	Maximumal tolerated dose of levodopa (+DCI) with anticholinergics and bromocriptine	Symptomatic treatment only
Senile parkinsonism (Diffuse cortical Lewy-body disease)	Levodopa with dicarboxylase inhibitor (DCI) in minimal dosage	Rising dose of levodopa with DCI	Maximal tolerated dose of levodopa and DCI	Symptomatic treatment only

DCI = decarboxylase inhibitor.

to prolong the action of levodopa. Selegiline may, therefore, be useful in some cases suffering severe "on-off" fluctuations of response to levodopa. Claims have been made that Selegiline may slow down the progression of the disease, but no conclusive evidence is currently available to support this possibility. Multi-centre trials are in progress.

Depression often requires specific antidepressant treatment with tricyclic or tetracyclic antidepressants, where their anticholinergic affects may be an added benefit. Monoamine oxidase A inhibitors cannot be used with levodopa.

Constipation is also a common problem for patients with parkinsonism. Management should be with increased fluid intake with meals and added bran or bulk-purgatives such as Fybogel or Isogel. A regular nightly dose of irritant laxative is often necessary in addition. Senna or bisacodyl are generally well tolerated.

Abnormal Movement Disorders: Dystonias

Dystonia

Generalised dystonia is rare in the elderly but focal dystonias are more common and often present formidable problems of management.

Spasmodic torticollis is easily mistaken for cervical spondylosis especially when the symptoms are of recent onset. Patients tend to emphasise the symptom of pain in the neck and the "spasmodic" – that is variable – nature of the deformity in the cervical region may be overlooked unless looked for. The cause of spasmodic torticollis is unknown but there is seldom any significant psychopathology and the disorder is accepted as organic. It usually progresses over a few months to a state where the head is tilted and rotated on the neck and tremor or irregular jerky movements are superimposed on the abnormal posture. A diagnostic feature, when present, is the ability of some patients to correct the posture by light pressure with their finger-tip on the chin or forehead.

In some patients the condition slowly progresses with increasing pain and deformity. In others the condition becomes static, usually within 3 years. And occasionally it remits after an illness lasting a few months. The treatment of spasmodic torticollis has been transformed by the introduction of botulinus toxin injection of the muscles. This method has proved superior to medical treatment with tetrabenazine, or high dose anticholinergic therapy (benzhexol up to 30–60mg/day introduced over 6 months). Injection of botulinus toxin into the anterior cervical muscles will usually relieve symptoms for 2–3 months. The injection has then to be repeated for a further few months' relief of the symptoms.

Idiopathic blephoraspasm, like spasmodic torticollis is another example of a focal dystonia, and may also progress over a period of months to a state where the patient is functionally blind during the spasms from active closure of the eyes. Botulinus toxin injection is generally safe and extremely effective but has to be repeated every 10–12 weeks. In those cases where treatment by injection is unacceptable, tetrabenazine may suppress the dystonia.

Writers cramp is considered in Chapter 10.

Facial Dyskinesia

Facial dyskinesia may develop as an idiopathic phenomenon or present as a complication of phenothiazine treatment – tardive dyskinesia. Parkinson's disease treated with levodopa often causes facial or generalised dyskinesia, and Huntington's chorea may present in the elderly with choreiform facial movements of this type. Treatment is with tetrabenazine, which will give relief in the majority of cases. However, this drug causes severe side effects and may not be tolerated in adequate dosage. Sedation and depression are common early symptoms (the latter sometimes controllable with additional antidepressant treatment). Parkinsonism tends to develop as a late side effect of tetrabenazine.

Dystonic Dysarthria

Dystonic dysarthria presents with a speech disorder where the flow of speech is interrupted by involuntary movements of the glottis, larynx and nasopharynx. Speech becomes jerky and explosive but the disorder seldom spreads to involve other muscles. Tetrabenazine, high dose benzhexol, and baclofen are occasionally helpful. Recurrent laryngeal nerve section has been recommended, but injection with botulinus toxin will probably become the accepted treatment.

9 Attacks of Loss of Consciousness and Disturbance of Memory

Consciousness is the state of awareness of self and surroundings and is normally associated with the recording of memory. Thus concussive head injury will lead initially to unrousable unconsciousness followed by a drowsy state where there is diminished awareness. Consciousness can only be said to have fully recovered after concussion when the patient is able to record continuous memory. The duration of loss of consciousness in concussion is measured by the time from the head injury to the recovery from post-traumatic amnesia, and the duration of post-traumatic amnesia correlates well with the severity of the head injury. Disturbance of consciousness may, therefore, be without any discernible drowsiness. But specific defects of memory – the amnesic states – should be classified separately from conditions causing disturbance of consciousness because they imply a focal disturbance of brain function. In this chapter we will consider the causes of blackouts and the amnesic states, since these are seen relatively commonly in the elderly population.

Attacks of Loss of Consciousness

Recurrent blackouts are among the commonest reasons for patients to present to their doctor or specialist. The attack itself is usually very alarming to the eye-witness (less so to the patient) and the implications in terms of possible cause, risk of injury and future care and independence create an urgency to the problem. The physician has to be fully equipped with, firstly, a plan of differential diagnosis; then the skill to elicit a detailed and comprehensive history (on which diagnosis usually depends) from patient and eye-witness; and finally knowledge of management relating to social matters and driving as well as medication. Special investigations are seldom crucial in the management of patients presenting in this way. They may confirm a clinical diagnosis, but occasionally an abnormal EEG or ECG will suggest a diagnosis which can be excluded on clinical grounds – some 10% of the population have abnormal

EEGs. The diagnosis must, therefore, be clinical and a normal ECG does not exclude cardiac dysrhythmia any more than a normal EEG excludes epilepsy.

Acute or recurrent confusional states are dealt with in Chapter 3 and are not considered here. In this chapter we are considering the patient who suffers attack(s) or episode(s) in which consciousness is impaired, and then recovers with no (or only minimal) persisting symptoms. This, then, is the differential diagnosis of epilepsy in the elderly.

Epilepsy is probably best defined as a condition where there is a tendency to fits or seizures; and fits come in a wide variety of manifestations which it would be beyond the scope of this book to consider in detail. But in the elderly many of the minor epilepsies are rare – for example, classical petit mal or myoclonic epilepsy. By contrast disturbances of cerebral perfusion are commoner than in the young and it must be admitted that many elderly patients with dizzy attacks defy diagnosis. Fortunately such cases usually cease to have attacks spontaneously or declare themselves by the evolution of the condition.

In terms of brain function, loss of consciousness implies either a disturbance of cerebral metabolism or a disturbance of the electrical activity of the brain. Some 65% of the blood glucose and 20% of the oxygen capacity of the blood is utilised at rest by the brain. General disturbance of cerebral perfusion will, therefore, lead to rapid loss of consciousness and may be caused by cardiac asystole, profound bradycardia, hypotension or sudden fall in cardiac output. Sudden loss of perfusion in the vertebro-basilar territory by embolic occlusion may give rise to transient loss or disturbance of consciousness. But carotid occlusion has to be associated with extensive and persisting hemisphere ischaemia before there is loss of consciousness. Carotid transient ischaemic attacks are, therefore, not normally associated with loss of consciousness.

Hypoglycaemic attacks are often difficult to diagnose; they constitute the only metabolic defect that presents a problem in differential diagnosis. Psychogenic attacks are less common in the old than earlier in life, but acute anxiety with or without hyperventilation and hysterical attention-seeking attacks are seen and may pose formidable problems of management. The successful diagnosis of such conditions is just the beginning of treatment and not the point at which the case can be dismissed as "functional". Thus panic attacks or hysterical seizures are more often symptomatic of a serious psychiatric disorder in the old than in the younger patient. Agitated depression is probably the commonest underlying cause and will often respond well to antidepressant treatment. The problem may be symptomatic of no more than a fear of some malignant disease and is a cry for medical investigation and reassurance.

The frequency and severity of epileptic attacks attributable to the primary epilepsies declines with advancing years, whereas cerebral infarctions, neoplasia and degenerative disorders associated with epilepsy all become more common in the old. Epilepsy should always be regarded as a symptom rather than a disease and never more so than in the elderly patient. However, epilepsy which is a symptom of brain tumour with clear-cut clinical features is not necessarily an indication for detailed radiological assessment since the demonstration of the tumour may not influence management. Epilepsy is commonly symptomatic of alcohol abuse or medication. Thus the onset of alcoholic dementia may be signalled by one or a series of epileptic fits. The water intoxication from large quantities of beer in someone with diminished renal function, or the acute effects of large quantities of alcohol may precipitate seizures. In this situation, however, the attribution to ethanol can only be made by exclusion of other possibilities, and careful investigation is, therefore, necessary. Similarly the withdrawal of sedative drugs, especially phenobarbitone or benzodiazepines, may precipitate seizures, and phenothiazines and tricyclics not uncommonly provoke epileptic attacks. By contrast, the elderly person is more resistant than the young to the epileptogenic effects of fever, sleep deprivation and head injury. Early post-traumatic epilepsy in the old should, therefore, raise the suspicion of an intracranial complication of head injury, and similarly the elderly person with a fever who suffers a fit should be investigated with intracranial sepsis in mind – meningitis or brain abscess.

History, Examination and Investigation

The correct diagnosis of the cause of a "blackout" nearly always depends on the history, but it is the account of the attack given by an eye-witness that contains the greatest information. The history should detail the circumstances of the attack, possible provocative factors and a detailed description of all symptoms leading up to the moment when consciousness is lost. The past medical history should record previous attacks, drug history, history of head injury or neurological illness. It should also record any medical history associated with occlusive vascular disease or hypertension, or neoplasia, and any antecedent history to suggest developing neurological disease, including dementia.

During the phase of unconsciousness an eye-witness account of convulsive movements, colour, and posture of the limbs should be elicited. Incontinence or tongue-biting classically suggest epilepsy and are rare in any attack that is psychologically determined. Any residual symptoms after consciousness is restored may indicate the nature and cause of the episode.

The examination of the patient should concentrate on:

1. Excluding papilloedema – indicative of raised intracranial pressure
2. Excluding signs of focal neurological deficit or dementia
3. Excluding signs suggesting cardiac arrhythmia or postural hypotension
4. Excluding signs of drug treatment (or withdrawal) or alcoholism as the cause for the attack

When the examination of the patient is complete, a working diagnosis must be arrived at because the subsequent management of the patient depends on it. Thus a number of questions must immediately be answered:

1. What investigations are appropriate?
2. What treatment should be recommended?
3. What special advice should be given with respect to risk of further attacks, activities to be avoided and, in the case of car drivers, medical fitness to drive?

Table 9.1. Causes of loss of consciousness in the elderly

Epilepsy
1. Primary (and usually lifelong)
2. Secondary to:
   a. Stroke: single or multiple
   b. Tumour: primary or metastatic; intrinsic or extrinsic
   c. Degenerative brain disorders: Alzheimer's disease
                                    Jakob–Creutzfeld disease
                                    Progressive multifocal leucoencephalopathy
   d. Drug induced: i by provocation, e.g., antidepressants, phenothiazines, alcohol
                    ii by withdrawal, e.g., benzodiazepines, barbiturates
   e. Intracranial sepsis: meningitis, abscess, subdural empyema
   f. Metabolic (see below)

Impaired cerebral perfusion
1. Physiological: vasovagal syncope especially after prolonged recumbency, or nutritional deprivation
2. Postural hypotension in autonomic neuropathy, multi-system atrophy, fixed reduced cardiac output (aortic stenosis, pericarditis), due to drugs (phenothiazines, hypotensives, diuretics, sedatives, tricyclices) Addisons' disease and hypopituitarism
3. Cardiac dysrrhythmias. paroxysmal atrial or ventricular flutter, fibrillation, heart block, sick-sinus syndrome
4. Others: micturition syncope, cough syncope, carotid sinus stimulation, profound anaemia, vertebro-basilar TIA, "drop attacks"

Psychogenic
1. Acute panic or phobic attacks with or without hyperventilation
2. "Hysterical"

Metabolic
1. Diabetic keto-acidosis
2. Hypoglycaemic
3. Hypothermic
4. Thiamine deficiency (Wernicke's encephalopathy)
5. Hepatic, uraemic, hypo- or hypercalcaemic

Epilepsy

Classical tonic-clonic seizures that have been witnessed seldom cause diagnostic difficulties but minor attacks with epileptic automatisms may be more difficult, especially where the family and patient have not realised the behaviour is episodic or paroxysmal.

Case 9.1

A retired 78-year-old schoolmaster was brought by his daughter who thought her father was dementing with loss of memory. He had become forgetful, losing his possessions in the house and occasionally failing to "take in" conversational remarks. The diagnosis was suspected clinically only when it became clear that most of the time he was lucid and alert but could confirm that he experienced "blank spells" when he felt "a little dizzy". Treatment with anticonvulsant drugs restored normal behaviour.

Table 9.2. Indications for CT scan in an elderly patient with epilepsy

Progressive neurological deficit
Focal aura, focal signs or focal EEG
Raised intracranial pressure
Frequency of seizures increasing in spite of optimal anticonvulsant treatment

Detailed discussion of the drug treatment of epilepsy is beyond the scope of this book but, in general, anticonvulsant drugs are well tolerated in the elderly, and cross reactions with other drugs are rare. Epilepsy is an absolute bar to driving until two years have elapsed from the date of the last day-time attack.

The majority of patients with epilepsy presenting in late life have a small cerebral infarct as the cause. But tumours – metastases, meningiomas and gliomas – may present in this way and chronic subdural haematoma is an occasional cause. Other structural lesions – benign cysts, aneurysms, angiomas, pituitary lesions and many others – may account for the single or recurrent epileptic episode. Nocturnal confusion or incontinence may be the presenting feature of epilepsy in old age and focal post-ictal paresis (Todd's paralysis) is frequently misdiagnosed in the elderly as stroke.

Epilepsy may be the presenting symptom of a dementia, intracranial sepsis or a metabolic disorder. And drugs may lead to an epileptic seizure either because they are potentially epileptogenic or because withdrawal of most sedatives may provoke fits (see Table 9.1).

In the elderly, epilepsy should be investigated with CT scan if there are associated signs or symptoms to suggest a progressive neurological abnormality, especially if there is suspicion of subdural haematoma. CT scans are also indicated when the seizures have a focal aura or there is a strongly focal EEG (and where the signs are not easily explicable by stroke), and where there are symptoms or signs of raised intracranial pressure or where the frequency of seizures is increasing in spite of optimal anticonvulsant treatment. Table 9.2 summarises the indications for CT scan in an elderly patient with epilepsy.

Cardiac Dysrrhythmias

Typically, the loss of consciousness is abrupt and without warning. The patient is ashen pale but with recovery of consciousness a sudden flushing of the face may occur. Some patients describe palpitations or chest discomfort immediately preceding the attack, and others note loss of vision before losing consciousness. It is useful to ask spouse or family to note the pulse and heart rate during an attack, where cardiac dysrrhythmia is suspected. Examination may show heart block or cardiac dysrrhythmia and the ECG may provide information confirming the clinical diagnosis, but continuous ECG monitoring may be required.

Postural Hypotension

Fainting is less common as a physiological phenomenon in the old than in the young and this fact presumably reflects the progressive loss of elasticity of the vascular system with age. But there are a number of neurological disorders that afflict the old and that may present with unconsciousness due to hypotension.

Drugs, especially sedatives, phenothiazines (sometimes prescribed for "dizziness" symptomatic of hypotension and thus exacerbating the symptom), antidepressants, diuretics and over-enthusiastic use of hypotensive agents are a potent cause of fainting. Parkinson's disease and the multi-system atrophies are commonly associated with low blood pressure. Autonomic neuropathy may be primary or part of a multi-system atrophy. It also occurs in diabetes and other peripheral neuropathies. Dehydration, anaemia, aortic stenosis (and other cardiac causes of fixed reduced cardiac output) are common general medical causes and, finally, the occasional case of Addison's disease or hypopituitarism must be borne in mind.

In the elderly patient a syncopal attack may commonly lack the characteristic autonomic prodromata seen in the young. Thus the patient may deny any symptoms of warning of the attack such as feeling stifled, hot, nauseated, dizzy or trembly. The onset may be abrupt and difficult to distinguish from other causes of loss of consciousness or falling.

Treatment of the patient with postural hypotension must start with the treatment of the cause where possible. But hypotension due to autonomic failure may be a difficult condition to treat effectively. It is a cause of much morbidity and is occasionally fatal. Salt supplements to the diet should be recommended in the mild case and fludrocortisone added if necessary. Compression stockings are often poorly tolerated and frequently do not help. Indomethacin has been reported to be useful in occasional cases.

Cough and Micturition Syncope

Any rise of intrathoracic pressure (as in the Valsalva manoeuvre) will lead to reduced venous return to the heart. If the patient is standing or sitting upright and if circumstances are conducive to low systemic blood pressure, this reduced venous return may cause a sharp fall in cardiac output leading to reduced cerebral perfusion and syncope.

A paroxysm of coughing in the heavy smoker is a typical example of this sequence of events and is usually called "cough syncope". The male patient who gets out of bed to pass water may have to strain slightly to initiate micturition and thereby induce a similar sequence of events – micturition syncope.

"Drop Attacks"

Attacks of unexplained falling with momentary or minimal loss of consciousness in the middle-aged or elderly subject (usually female) may defy diagnosis and qualify for the descriptive title "drop attacks". The implication of this diagnosis is a good prognosis and it, therefore, follows that the diagnosis should only be made in retrospect when the attacks have ceased. Many patients presenting in this way prove later to have epilepsy, cardiac dysrhythmias or other causes for their attacks and diagnosis is occasionally delayed by the reassuringly simple description "drop attacks".

Case 9.2

This obese 64-year-old female presented with the complaint of repeated falling and damage to her thighs and knees. The falling was without any warning and she was able immediately to pick herself up and continue what she was doing. A diagnosis of "benign drop attacks" was reviewed when the attacks continued without any spontaneous improvement. The only diagnostic clue, a tachycardia, finally proved to be indicative of thyrotoxicosis and we eventually concluded that her drop attacks had been caused by a proximal thyrotoxic myopathy.

Vertebro-basilar Ischaemia

The concept of embolic disturbance of perfusion of the brainstem through sudden transitory occlusion of the vertebro-basilar system has been popular since the 1950s, possibly because it is usually unprovable as a diagnosis. It is probably rare, but may be seriously entertained as a diagnosis if loss of consciousness is preceded or followed by symptoms or signs of brainstem nuclear disturbance or long-tract abnormalities. Thus diplopia, nystagmus, oral or pharyngeal paraesthesiae, intense vertigo and paraesthesiae of the body and limbs, especially if associated with tetraparetic signs, may support the diagnosis. Treatment is with anti-embolic therapy but the prognosis is surprisingly good. If there is not hypertension, anticoagulants may be considered.

The clinical features of subclavian steal with blood pressure 15 mm Hg (or more) greater in one arm than the other will suggest innominate or subclavian artery occlusion or stenosis with reversed flow in one vertebral artery and reduced perfusion of the brainstem. This condition will more often cause transitory brainstem symptoms than loss of consciousness. Attacks induced by vigorous activity involving the arms are probably so rare as to be almost mythical.

Post-stroke "Narcolepsy" and Drowsiness

Some patients after recent stroke exhibit fluctuations in consciousness which are important to recognise, as failure to do so may lead to the unwarranted assumption that the patient is so damaged after the stroke that functional recovery is unlikely. The patient may be identified by nursing or rehabilitation staff as being drowsy or unable to co-operate with physiotherapy or occupational therapy. In the most extreme form the patient may be observed apparently to fall asleep in the middle of doing something (for example, while being walked by the physiotherapist) and to be extremely difficult to arouse for some time afterwards. In such cases there are no features suggestive of an epileptic seizure. The patient may wake up equally suddenly. Other patients with seemingly lesser degrees of the same condition show variation in level of arousal over the course of several hours or days. In most patients with this disorder of consciousness, treatment with dexamphetamine restores a level of consciousness compatible with full co-operation. In some patients the result of giving dexamphetamine is dramatic, an otherwise moribund stroke victim being transformed within a day into someone who is more or less fully mobile and independent. Treatment with dexamphetamine (the drug always being administered first thing in the morning in order to prevent disruption of sleep at night) is usually started at a dose of 2.5 mg, the dose being increased, if necessary, every two to three days up to a maximum of 10 mg each day until a satisfactory response has been achieved. A trial without the drug should take place two weeks after the maximum therapeutic effect is reached: most patients do not relapse with a diminished level of consciousness at this stage, but those who do should be treated at the optimum dose for a further month. At the end of this period it is very unusual for the drug to be required any further. Habituation to dexamphetamine does not seem to occur when it is used in this condition.

Cataplexy seldom presents in old age.

Hypothermia

When body temperature falls below about 32 °C there is usually some degree of impairment of consciousness going on to coma. Exposure to low temperatures, under-nutrition, alcohol, or sedative drugs may all lead to the development of hypothermia, which is particularly common in the elderly. Hypoglycaemia, myxoedema, hypopituitarism or even cachexia with profoundly reduced muscle mass are rarer causes.

The clinical features include pallor of the skin, absence of shivering, and a change in the consistency of subcutaneous tissue with a rigidity of muscle tone. The tendon reflexes are usually preserved, but may show the slow "tonic" relaxation of the patient with myxoedema. The pupils are typically constricted. The diagnosis is made by recording body temperature but a low-reading thermometer must be used because the standard clinical thermometer does not register temperatures below 35 °C. Treatment is by the slow re-warming of the patient with gentle external heat and the administration of warm sweetened drinks.

Amnesic States

Clinical tests of memory are designed to make distinctions between (i) immediate recall, (ii) recent memory and (iii) remote memory. These distinctions are of more than academic importance because they usefully separate the three categories of amnesic states. Thus, patients with mild disturbance of consciousness, where it may be difficult clinically to discern that the patient is drowsy or obtunded, may show abnormality on tests of immediate recall, because the recording of memory is dependent on attention. Tests such as digit retention may be used. The patient is asked to repeat back a series of numbers, either in the order dictated or in reverse order. Six or seven digits forwards and four or five digits backwards is an acceptable "normal". A defect of immediate recall suggests either a slight impairment of consciousness and attention or a lack of motivation which may, of course, amount to a hysterical or psychogenic amnesia.

Abnormalities of recent memory are characteristic of focal pathology affecting the hypothalamus or upper brainstem in the peri aqueductal region, or lesions involving both hippocampi in the temporal lobes. Thus classically alcoholic amnesic states (Korsakoff's syndrome) and patients with severe nutritional disorders, as well as those who have suffered prolonged vomiting, may exhibit the characteristic memory defect. Bilateral temporal lobe lesions affecting the hippocampi and occasionally seen following bilateral stroke in the posterior cerebral territory may also give rise to this form of memory disturbance.

The patient, while alert and able to perform normally in tests of immediate recall, fails on tests where there is an interval between the event or information given and the recall of the information. Thus a "five minute name, address and flower test" where seven items of information are given, may reveal abnormality (see Chap. 3).

Remote memory is tested by asking the patient about past events – the dates of the World Wars or the names of the Queen's children. An isolated defect of remote memory suggests a disturbance of the long-term memory storage system and in the presence of normal recent memory a defect of remote memory suggests a diffuse cerebral disorder such as Alzheimer's disease (see Chap. 3).

Wernicke's Encephalopathy and Korsakoff's Psychosis

Deficiencies of vitamins of the B group are common in the elderly. Chronic malnutrition is regularly seen even in advanced western countries, as the product of impaired standards of self-care, especially in the male following bereavement, or in the context of poverty, alcoholism, or social isolation. Memory impairment along with depression, lassitude and weakness are seen in vitamin deficiency involving all the B group. In nicotinic acid deficiency (pellagra) stomatitis, diarrhoea and skin pigmentation are also seen. But it is in thiamine deficiency that there is the most devastating affect on memory.

"Wernicke's encephalopathy" and "Korsakoff's psychosis" respectively describe the acute and chronic manifestations of thiamine deficiency. Although alcoholism is by far the most important aetiological factor, chronic malnutrition especially associated with vomiting or upper gastro-intestinal tract disorder may cause this condition.

Wernicke's encephalopathy presents as an acute medical emergency with a triad of ataxia, ophthalmoplegia and confusion which on examination (and in patients where testing is possible) proves to be characterised by severe recent memory defect. The ataxia has the features of a cerebellar disorder with associated nystagmus but there is little or no dysarthria. It is easy to mistake these cases for posterior fossa lesion and the normal CT scan then leaves a diagnostic vacuum.

Features of peripheral neuropathy (arreflexia, glove/stocking hypaesthesia) may suggest that the ataxia is due to a sensory neuropathy.

Mental changes in the milder case may consist only of apathy and depression, progressing to impairment of consciousness. The profound disorder of memory may be concealed behind a facade of irrelevant chatter or give the appearance of an agitated, confusional state. Confabulation is a characteristic feature so that the patient may fill defects in their memory with a wealth of imaginary detail. There is seldom any insight by the patient of their memory defect. Specific tests of memory should always be attempted where Korsakoff's mental state is a possibility. The patient is nearly always disorientated in time. Recent events either of current affairs or in personal experience cannot be recalled. And current memorising of a short story or "name, address and flower test" is reduced in the severe case to nil. Terrifying visual hallucinations may provoke the patient into a state of severe agitation requiring heavy sedation with a drug such as chlorpromazine, or diazepam.

In the advanced case a combination of confusion, weakness and impairment of consciousness may make the diagnosis extremely difficult. Thus ataxia, sensory tests, eye signs and tests of memory all become impossible to elicit and in such a case empirical treatment with thiamine should always be given after blood has been taken for estimation of thiamine levels or transketolase activity.

Transient Global Amnesia

This condition is not uncommon, but is poorly recognised. This is unfortunate because the condition inevitably causes considerable anxiety amongst relatives as well as in the patient and if it is not recognised to be the benign disorder that it is, these anxieties will not be laid to rest.

The syndrome of transient global amnesia is characterised by a solitary attack (or a few attacks) of profound memory disturbance with no loss of alertness or insight. The attack is of abrupt onset, lasts usually between one and twelve hours and the patient recovers leaving no sequelae. During the attack the patient is aware of his (for the condition affects males more often than females) amnesia and repeatedly asks the same question "where am I?", "What am I doing here?", etc. But he is unable to recall information given during the attack nor to recall past events. Patients look bewildered and anxious but, surprisingly, learnt skills are not impaired so that these patients commonly drive their cars safely, can read and write normally and are able, for example, to play musical instruments during the attack with their accustomed skill. Remote memories are usually preserved so the patient has no loss of personal identity and can identify friends and relations, although he may be unclear why they are in his company at that time.

The attack terminates less abruptly than its onset but within half an hour the patient is recording information accurately and is able to describe the events that immediately preceded the onset of the global amnesia.

The mechanism of the condition is unknown, but transient ischaemia in the vertebro-basilar territory is generally considered the explanation in the majority of cases. However, a mechanism of this sort scarcely explains what is an important feature of the condition, namely its tendency to be a single isolated episode never to be repeated. Similarly there may be no features of cerebro-vascular disease and no increased future risk of stroke. It is, therefore, justified to give an optimistic prognosis.

Familiarity with the clinical features described should leave the diagnosis beyond doubt and distinguish cases of transient global amnesia from epilepsy, hypoglycaemia (where behaviour is usually abnormal), acute intoxications, or psychogenic states.

Amnesia in Diffuse Cerebral Disorder

The acute disturbances of higher mental function (acute confusional states) may show a pronounced disturbance of memory but usually this is associated with some impairment of consciousness and attention. The post-traumatic amnesia would be the typical example. Amnesia as part of a dementing process typically affects memory diffusely, involving remote as well as recent memory. In the early stages of a dementing process much of the recent memory impairment may seem to be part of a failure to attend or concentrate. "Granny is only forgetful because she doesn't listen" is a frequent comment.

Alzheimer's disease and multi-infarct dementia typically show severe defects of remote memory whereas the dementia of frontal lobe type and the dementia of progressive supra-nuclear palsy may show very few amnesic features.

10 Loss of Use in the Upper Limb

The complaint of disturbance of function in the arm may signify a wide range of disorders and diagnosis is frequently difficult, especially in the elderly. Many important principles of neurological examination are exemplified by patients presenting in this way and this chapter has been used to discuss a variety of conditions, ranging from dystonias to mononeuropathies and from "frozen shoulder" to the Eaton–Lambert syndrome.

Although neurological disturbance usually accounts for the symptoms, arthropathy may complicate the clinical picture. Most elderly patients attribute any disturbance of use in the arm or hand to "arthritis" often referring to an X-ray examination of their neck as proof of the diagnosis of "arthritis of the spine". Caution should be exercised before this explanation is accepted because degenerative changes in the neck on X-ray films are practically universal and very often a neurological disorder is the basis of the symptoms.

Case 10.1
A 72-year-old male had been attending a physiotherapy department for some months with the complaint of pain in the shoulder attributed to "arthritis" – probably of the cervical spine since the patient was undergoing intermittent traction of the neck. His pain improved rapidly as soon as his Parkinson's disease was treated.

Painful restriction of movement at a joint is the hallmark of an arthropathy but the distinction of pain due to arthropathy and pain from other causes is complicated by the fact that in old age two or more conditions frequently co-exist. The patient's description of her pain may not be very helpful since it is seldom easy for a patient to distinguish between the quality or site of referred or local pain. Furthermore, for reasons that are poorly understood, pain tends to radiate widely in the arm: the pain of carpal tunnel syndrome is a good example.

The History

In taking a history from a patient presenting with loss of use in the hand or arm, concentrate first on discovering the extent and severity of weakness. Is the patient able to move the shoulder – to brush her hair or reach behind her back? Is the elbow weak, for lifting the hand to the mouth, for instance, or is the triceps weak in the "pushing" movement of rising from a chair; and, perhaps most importantly, is grip or fine movement in the hand affected, with loss of dexterity? Is there difficulty with fastening buttons, shoelaces, zips? Can the grip support the weight of a loaded basket?

"Weakness". Neuropathic weakness of the arm must be separated into the upper motor neurone or lower motor neurone type by attention to a few points in the history and examination. With spastic weakness of the arm (upper motor neurone) the patient describes the limb as "heavy", "dead", "as if it doesn't belong to me", whereas words like "weak", "floppy", "useless" are more likely to be applied in flaccid weakness. Parkinson's disease symptoms develop slowly and patients are usually impressed by the slowness of hand movement and loss of dexterity (especially for writing) and the inability to perform sustained rhythmical movements such as polishing furniture or brushing their teeth. The affected limb does not swing during walking. Apparent "weakness" may result from pain – from whatever source – from loss of position sense and from conditions associated with dystonia such as writer's cramp.

Secondly, sensory disturbance should be enquired about. Does part or all of the hand feel numb or tingly? Does the patient drop things involuntarily?

Finally, enquire about positive symptoms – pain and, equally important, paraesthesiae because the latter are more likely to be distributed more precisely in the territory of a dermatome or peripheral nerve. Positive motor symptoms such as tremor or abnormal involuntary movements will usually be evident without specific enquiry, but occasionally an episodic involuntary movement will indicate a focal epileptic disorder.

In summary, the history consists of information relating simply to three things – disturbance of function or weakness, sensory loss and paraesthesiae, and pain.

The Examination

The examination of the patient with loss of use in the arm is all-important and must be conducted with a differential diagnosis in mind. Neurological disorders affecting the arm follow recognisable patterns determined by the neuroanatomy. Where a root lesion is suspected, all the muscles supplied by that nerve root should be tested and compared with the other side; tests of cutaneous sensation in the same segmental dermatome should follow. But where a peripheral nerve lesion is suspected, the muscles supplied by that nerve should be tested and similarly sensory loss for that nerve mapped out. Thus the examination should always concentrate on those physical signs most likely to give the diagnostic information. A "routine" neurological examination (like "routine enquiry") will result in much useless information from which it may be impossible to come to any diagnostic conclusion. Always remember that the aim is to reach a diagnosis and assessment of your patient's disability.

Loss of use in the hand may result from upper or lower motor neurone weakness, extra pyramidal disease, sensory loss (especially posterior column) or abnormal involuntary movements including tremor; or it may result from muscle pain with or without myopathic weakness or joint pain, either focal or generalised.

There are some patterns of symptomatology affecting the upper limb where the history is so characteristic that there is little diagnostic difficulty: carpal tunnel syndrome, tennis elbow and frozen shoulder are examples. And the patient with stroke involving the lower limb as well as the arm, or the patient with other clinical features of *Herpes zoster* or Parkinson's disease, may pose little diagnostic difficulty. But usually there will be a differential diagnosis and a firm opinion and plan of management can only be reached after careful examination.

The Signs

Inspection
Inspection of the limb involves careful comparison with the opposite side. Generally it is easier to pick up muscle-wasting by inspection than by measurement. Compare the shoulder girdle, triceps muscles (crossing the arms across the chest or holding the shoulders in partial abduction) and scrutinise all the small hand muscles on palmar and dorsal aspects. Wherever there is the possibility of motor neurone disease look long and hard for fasciculation – it may provide the diagnosis which can then be confirmed by excluding sensory signs or bladder disturbance.

Tone
Muscle tone is an important physical sign and is best elicited by quick jerky movements to the relaxed limb, especially flexion/extension of elbow and wrist, and pronation/supination of the forearm. The typical "clasp knife" spastic hypertonia may be present in the wrist in cervical cord lesions as well as in hemisphere lesions. Rigid hypertonia of the "lead pipe" variety may be a vital clue to early Parkinson's disease.

In many elderly patients, especially those with cerebral arteriosclerosis, there is an inability to relax the limb for testing muscle tone. Even when their attention is diverted the arm is held sunny as soon as it is picked up. "Paratonia" of this type should raise the possibility of generalised cerebral changes and grasp reflexes, palmo-mental reflexes and pouting reflexes may be positive (see p. 10, Chap. 1). These signs may have lateralising significance in a unilateral frontal lesion.

Power
Muscle power cannot be reliably tested in the presence of pain – even when the pain is independent of movement at the relevant joint. But where pain is not a problem, power should be tested methodically through a representative range of muscles for two reasons; to define the group of muscles involved in terms of their innervation (i.e., are all the muscles that are weak supplied by, for example, the T1 root or the ulnar nerve?); and to assess the severity of weakness at that time so that subsequent comparisons of improvement or deterioration can be made.

Thus, in upper neurone weakness of the arm the distribution will be "pyramidal" – that is affecting abduction of the shoulder, the triceps and extension of the wrist; in a lower motor neurone weakness the muscles involved will form a pattern depending on the nerve damaged – so that abduction of the shoulder and flexion of the elbow in a C5/6 lesion; thenar muscle weakness in a median neuropathy – with or without forearm muscle involvement depending on the site of the lesion. And weakness of all the intrinsic hand muscles sparing the thenar group where the ulnar nerve is damaged.

Thoracic Outlet Syndromes (Including Pancoast tumours) tend to involve the abductor pollicis brevis preferentially, with early wasting and weakness. In these cases sensory loss over the inside of the forearm (in C8 T1 dermatomes) is easily overlooked. Wasting of all the intrinsic muscles of the hand may signify motor neurone disease or a T1 root lesion, but in the latter an ipsilateral Horner's syndrome may be found – if looked for.

Wasting and weakness of the hand but sparing the thenar muscles is characteristic of ulnar neuropathy. Ulnar lesions may occur at the elbow or wrist. An ulnar nerve lesion at the elbow will tend to involve flexor carpi ulnaris (with wasting of the ulnar border of the forearm and weakness of ulnar deviation of the wrist) and flexor digitorum profundus to the little and ring fingers. At the wrist an ulnar nerve lesion may involve only the superficial palmar branch when the only muscle involved will be abductor digiti minimi (but with prominent sensory symptoms and signs), or the deep palmar branch may be involved with extensive intrinsic muscle weakness and wasting without sensory loss. There is commonly some difficulty in assessing whether the ulnar nerve is thickened or abnormally tethered in an elderly patient and palpation of the nerve at the elbow may suggest a lesion at that level where examination of the neurological signs will suggest otherwise. Nerve conduction studies are valuable in defining the level of the lesion and also in providing a base line for future comparison. Thus the normal indications for surgical treatment of an ulnar nerve lesion should be restricted to progressive neurological deficit or pain. No recovery of function can be expected after surgery to the ulnar nerve if the lesion is long-standing and non-progressive.

Neuralgic amyotrophy presents with severe continuous pain deep in the shoulder, which resolves slowly after about 3 weeks. The pain is sufficient to disturb sleep and resists simple analgesia. The diagnosis can only be made by detecting wasting and weakness of scapular muscles (often with winging of the scapula). The finding of sensory loss confined to the circumflex nerve territory is useful confirmation of the diagnosis (that is sensory loss in an area about two inches in diameter over the insertion of deltoid). The prognosis is good with spontaneous resolution of pain within about 3 weeks and gradual recovery of power over about 18 months.

Herpes zoster affecting the nerve roots to the upper limb may occasionally affect the motor root as well as the sensory root. The prognosis for recovery from the resulting weakness is poor and is probably unaffected by oral acyclovir therapy. Evidence of motor root (or CNS) involvement by *Herpes zoster* is, therefore, an indication for the use of intravenous acyclovir.

Trauma or entrapment accounts for the majority of peripheral nerve lesions but vasculitic causes or diabetes account for a significant minority of cases in the elderly. Testing the urine for glucose and a blood count and ESR are the essential minimum investigations required.

Myopathic weakness affecting the upper limb will usually present with gener-alised symptoms – diffuse muscle and joint pain in polymyalgia rheumatica or polymyositis or bilateral muscle weakness also affecting the eye muscles and face in myasthenia gravis, and the lower limbs in Eaton–Lambert syndrome. But the case that is difficult to diagnose is where weakness from these causes is focal, affecting one arm or shoulder. If the diagnosis is made before the disease becomes generalised the patient may be saved many weeks or months of disability.

The tendon reflexes may be the clue to an upper motor neurone monoplegia where otherwise a brachial neuritis would be suspected.

The distinction between stroke and cerebral tumour presenting with loss of use in the arm should be made on the basis of history of onset, evolution of the symptoms and associated signs. The patient with stroke suffers the sudden or rapid onset of weakness which subsequently improves. Deterioration, if it does occur, tends to be "stepwise". A cerebral tumour will be characterised by the gradual insidious onset of symptoms which tend to progress slowly. With a tumour there may develop the signs and symptoms of raised intracranial pressure. Upper limb monoparesis from either cause is often associated with dysphasia if the right arm is involved or visual field deficit on the same side as the paresis.

Cord lesions in the upper or mid cervical region may be "extrinsic" and result from traumatic injury or degenerative changes in the cervical vertebrae, from compressive lesions such as subluxation of the atlanto-axial joint in rheumatoid arthritis or extradural abscess or metastases, or from "intrinsic" lesions of the cord especially glioma or syringomyelia. Extrinsic lesions rarely present with unilateral upper limb monoplegia but, rather, tend to cause paraparesis with or without pain in the neck and shoulder. Intrinsic lesions may present only with arm symptoms. When these are of pain and temperature loss with preservation of light touch and position sense, the diagnosis of syringomyelia is usually easily made. But any intrinsic cord lesion may give "dissociated sensory loss" of this type. Involvement of anterior horn cells may cause focal wasting, sometimes with fasciculation. Loss of tendon jerks in the arm is an important and almost invariable sign in syringomyelia. Continuous "boring" pain in the shoulder and arm is a common complaint in patients with intrinsic cord lesions of this type.

In cervical spondylotic myelopathy at C5/6, "inversion" of the radial reflex may be diagnostic. Tapping the radial head with a patella hammer fails to elicit a supinator jerk but causes finger flexion. This sign may be associated with reduced or absent biceps jerk and increased triceps and finger jerks. Brisk jerks in the presence of severe muscle wasting is suggestive of motor neurone disease. Absent jerks in one or both arms should suggest the possibility of multiple root lesions, syringomyelia, or Eaton–Lambert syndrome.

Arthropathic "weakess" is always associated with pain, which tends to be the foremost complaint of the patient. Even where the patient has a hemiplegic stroke a complicating painful "shoulder-hand" syndrome will be given greater emphasis than the weakness. Acute cervical disc prolapse, analogous to sciatica, presents with 'wry neck' and pain in the shoulder or arm. The pain may be severe and is exacerbated by any movement of the neck, so the head is often held in an abnormal posture. Pain, weakness and sensory symptoms referred to the arm suggests nerve root involvement as described above. Immobilisation of the neck in a collar and intermittent traction will usually lead to relief of all symptoms within a few weeks but the pain may require regular analgesia throughout this period.

Occasionally, persisting pain, often with paraesthesiae and sensory loss, indicates continuing irritation of the nerve root. If conservative measures fail, such cases may require surgical exploration of the affected root with decompression and facetectomy. But beware the occasional case of malignant disease with extradural or bone deposits.

Apparent paralysis of the shoulder, with muscle wasting, may result from an acute capsulitis of the shoulder. These cases are commonly referred to the neurological clinic but the limb is normal neurologically, apart from the muscles surrounding the shoulder joint where there is painful restriction of movement, particularly abduction and internal rotation. Occasionally the pain may only affect a narrow arc of movement on abduction, and this suggests inflammation of the tendon of the long head of biceps.

Chronic arthritic changes from gout, rheumatoid arthritis or osteoarthritis may all present with localised loss of use in the arm. Thus an acute flare-up of gout or rheumatoid arthritis affecting the elbow, wrist or shoulder may raise the suspicion of stroke. Equally, arthropathy of the elbow or wrist may be associated with ulnar or median neuropathy respectively, and the "tennis elbow" syndrome of inflammation of the common extensor tendon may cause symptoms and occasionally signs of radial neuropathy. These secondary neuropathies generally recover as the inflammatory process settles. Only in the case of median neuropathy associated with arthritis of the wrist is it commonly necessary to advise surgical decompression of the nerve.

Traumatic neuropathies are common in old age in certain particular circumstances or situations. The old lady who slips and falls backwards suffering "whiplash" injury to the neck may suffer acute trauma to the spinal cord and nerve roots in the neck. In such a case it is of the first importance to discover by appropriate X-ray examinations whether the vertebral column is intact and stable. Secondly, extrinsic compressive lesions should be excluded (haematoma, acute disc prolapse, bony fragments). Bruising of the cord (central cord syndrome) in such a case is characterised by paraparesis, mid cervical motor signs, dissociated sensory loss and very often by stinging or burning paraesthesiae in a "cape" distribution over the shoulders. In these cases, where the damage is not so severe as to require surgical intervention, the outcome is often good.

Dislocation of the shoulder is a commoner cause of brachial plexus injury in the elderly than are traction injuries. Elbow crutches, Zimmer frames and sticks all cause median neuropathy from pressure on the median nerve at the wrist. The superficial palmar branch of the ulnar nerve may also be compressed against the hook of the hamate bone. Padding of the grip on these appliances is seldom satisfactory in reversing such a neuropathy. Special moulded handles for crutches and sticks are available and are more satisfactory. Colles fracture of the radius may damage the median nerve and fractures of the humerus, which are also relatively common in the elderly, may cause a radial palsy. The prognosis for eventual recovery in these cases is good but it must be remembered that all peripheral nerve regrows at the rate of about 1 mm per day. Therefore injury to the radial nerve in the spiral groove of the humerus will take at least 200 days to recover.

"Numbness"

In many conditions sensation is involved along with motor disturbance, but occasionally sensory loss in the upper limb is the only sign of a neurological lesion. It is useful, therefore, to separate those conditions where sensory disturbance is prominent and where the sensory signs are of particular importance in diagnosis.

Sensory examination always depends on the patient's active co-operation, so that any patient who is obtunded, irritable or inattentive will give unreliable responses to sensory examination. Likewise, sensory examination should not be attempted where the patient is demented.

The first stage of any sensory examination must be to obtain the patient's attention and co-operation. At each stage these features should be reinforced and the aim of the particular test explained so that the patient understands what you are trying to discover. If the patient (or examiner) becomes tired, attention flags and the sensory signs become unreliable. This may mean that sensory examination has to be abbreviated and returned to later.

In the younger patient hysterical disturbances of arm function are not uncommon – particularly after trauma or in the context of psychiatric illness or litigation, but "functional" abnormalities of sensation are much less common in old age. Variability of sensory signs at this age is more likely, therefore, to be due to observer error or defects in technique of examination.

Table 10.1. Classification of causes for loss of use in the upper limb

	Weakness	
Neuropathic	*Myopathic*	*Arthropathic*
Upper motor neurone		
Stroke	Polymalgia rheumatica	Cervical spondylosis with referred root pain
Cerebral tumour	Polymyositis	Capsulitis of shoulder
High cervical cord lesion	Myasthenia gravis	
Chronic subdural haematoma	Eaton–Lambert syndrome	Osteoarthritis or rheumatoid arthritis of elbow, wrist or fingers
Extrapyramidal –		
Parkinson's disease		Gout
Lower motor neurone		
Motor neurone disease		
Cervical spondylotic radiculopathy		
Neuralgic amyotrophy		
Post-herpetic motor neuropathy		
Malignancy involving brachial plexus		
Mononeuropathies		
Entrapment		
Diabetic		
Vasculitic		
Trauma		
Peripheral neuropathy		

	"Numbness"	
Central		*Peripheral*
Parietal cortex		Nerve roots C5–T1
Stroke		
Tumour		
Thalamic		Thoracic outlet
High cervical cord lesions		Brachial plexus
		Peripheral nerve
		Radial
		Median
		Ulnar

Abnormal movements
Tremor
Benign "senile" essential tremor
Parkinson's disease
Cerebellar
Choreo-athetosis
Dystonia and Dyspraxia

The sensory examination concludes the neurological examination of the upper limb. It comes, therefore, at a stage when both patient and doctor may be tired. But the advantage of examining for sensory signs at the end of the physical examination is that by that stage the doctor should have a short differential diagnosis and thus be able to concentrate on those sensory signs that he knows will be especially relevant in confirming or refuting his diagnosis.

It is a waste of time to carry out detailed testing of sensation in the hand when the patient has a hemiplegia. It is essential to examine for cutaneous sensory loss over the inside of the forearm in a patient with Horner's syndrome, and to be certain of the precise cutaneous sensory loss where a median or ulnar neuropathy is suspected.

Some patients are over-helpful and report every nuance of subjective sensory change. The result can be hopelessly confusing. In such cases it is useful:

1. To compare the sensory changes in the two arms
2. To use "objective" tests of sensation so that the patient is asked to repeat "blunt" or "sharp" according to whether the skin is touched with a pencil or pin: or she is asked to report each time she perceived a light cotton-wool touch – failure to report suggesting loss of sensation; or test for two-point discrimination with special dividers or, if these are not available, a bent paper-clip so that the ends are 3–5 mm apart. In the elderly two points should be clearly and accurately perceived on the finger-tips when the separation is less than 5 mm

From the symptomatology and the motor examination the localisation of the lesion or disease process will already be suspected. Sensory testing should therefore be carried out bearing in mind:

1. *Cortical sensory defects* results from lesions in the parietal lobe. Primary sensation is usually preserved – touch, pain, vibration. But position sense, two-point discrimination, tactile localisation and graphaesthesia are characteristically lost. (Testing graphaesthesia involves writing numbers on the palm with a blunt point and asking the patient to identify the number by feel.) Sensory inattention (where the patient perceives a tactile or pain stimulus when it is applied to one limb but not when it is simultaneously applied to the opposite limb) is characteristic of parietal sensory loss.

2. *Thalamic lesions* or lesions in the upper brainstem may produce total hemi-anaesthesia on the side opposite to the lesion. When such sensory loss includes postural loss, it causes severe loss of function in the arm. But less severe thalamic lesions may cause the characteristic intractable thalamic pain with only slight impairment of temperature and pain sensation and no disturbance of function.

3. *Lesions of the lateral medulla* may give pain/temperature loss in the opposite arm, trunk and leg with ipsilateral pain/temperature loss in the face.

4. *Cord lesions* give bilateral loss of all modalities of sensation below a definite level. The spinal cord lesion cannot be situated below this level but may be several segments above it. The upper sensory level should always be defined precisely in a cord lesion at the highest level of subjective alteration of any modality as the most reliable indication of the level of the lesion. Dermatomes do not necessarily correspond to vertebral levels so that in the lumbar and low thoracic regions the vertebral level is four segments above the dermatome; in the upper thoracic region it is three and in the neck two segments above the corresponding vertebra.

5. *Intrinsic or hemicord lesions* may give "dissociated sensory loss" where loss of pain sensation is not associated with any corresponding loss of touch or position sense. In syringomyelia the hand may be anaesthetic for pain and temperature, but touch and position sense (and hence function) in the hand is normal. In the Brown–Sequard hemicord lesion, pain and temperature loss in one hand (and below) will be accompanied by loss of proprioception on the opposite side.

For reasons that are poorly understood, high cervical cord lesions (above C4) affecting the posterior columns may give a dissociated loss of position sense in the arm (with preservation of pain and temperature) which is also "suspended" – that is, confined to the arm and not affecting the legs.

6. *Root lesions* give sensory loss to all modalities in the dermatome of that segmental nerve root.

7. *In peripheral mononeuropathies* the distribution of the sensory loss is that of the nerve involved. Although all modalities will tend to be affected, there may be some "dissociation" due to a differential pathological effect on the larger myelinated (proprioceptive) fibres compared with the small unmyelinated pain/temperature fibres.

Mononeuropathic symptoms in the elderly fall naturally into two groups. There are the entrapment neuropathies where compression of the peripheral nerve occurs at specific (usually bony) points. Thus the lower trunks of the brachial plexus may be compressed by a cervical rib at the thoracic outlet. The ulnar nerve may be compressed in the medial condylar groove or at the wrist where it crosses the hook of the hamate. The radial nerve may be compressed against the humerus in the middle of the arm; or at the elbow as it passes into the forearm. And, finally, the median nerve may be entrapped as it enters the forearm beneath pronator teres or, most commonly, at the wrist in the carpal tunnel.

The other group of mononeuropathies are those associated with a vascular systemic disorder. Thus, diabetes may present with wrist drop through a radial palsy or a mononeuropathy affecting the ulnar nerve. Collagen vascular disease, especially polyarteritis nodosa, and rheumatoid arthritis, are often the cause of symptoms of this type.

8. In generalised *peripheral neuropathies* the longest sensory fibres tend to be affected most so that a "glove and stocking" distribution of anaesthesia will result and the legs will be affected as well as the arms. In such cases the tendon reflexes are normally lost and the "level" of sensory loss is somewhat indefinite.

Where a peripheral neuropathy is suspected, it is important to palpate peripheral nerves for thickening. The ulnar nerve and terminal branches of the radial and anterior tibial nerves can be examined in this way and compared for normality, if necessary, with the examiner's own. Hypertrophy of peripheral nerve suggests either abnormal infiltration or deposition in the perineurium (as in leprosy or amyloid disease) or a chronic demyelinating peripheral neuropathy.

Abnormal Involuntary Movements

Tremor

Tremor is defined as a regular rhythmical oscillating movement which is so common as to be regarded as one of the characteristics of old age. This common form of tremor – senile essential tremor – must be clearly distinguished from Parkinson's disease tremor (see Chap. 8), because it is not associated with the other features of that condition and does not respond to specific anti-parkinsonian drugs.

Senile essential tremor is normally absent if the limb is at complete rest but it may be difficult to obtain the complete relaxation of the muscles that is necessary to suppress the tremor. A sustained posture – for example, when the arms are held out in front of the patient – will exacerbate the tremor and it will persist during voluntary movement. For these reasons senile tremor is not only a source of embarrassment and distress, it also can be the cause of considerable disability.

In some patients essential tremor develops long before old age but it tends to progress more noticeably after the age of 60 years. While the hands are often severely affected, jaw, larynx and neck are also commonly involved.

Most patients derive some temporary improvement in this tremor from alcohol in quantities much too small to induce inebriation. Those who have not discovered this effect of alcohol may need reassurance that it is a safe form of symptomatic treatment and unlikely to lead to alcoholism if it is used only when essential. Beta-blockers (such as propranolol) may reduce the tremor by as much as 30% but side effects are not well tolerated in the very elderly. Primidone may be helpful in some cases. The occasional severe case, where symptoms are predominantly unilateral and there are no features of cerebro-vascular disease, may be considered for stereo-tactic thalamotomy.

The tremor of Parkinson's disease is discussed in Chapter 8. Cerebellar ataxia may be accompanied by severe tremor, particularly when deriving from damage to the brain stem or red nucleus. This is seen most commonly in the younger patient with multiple sclerosis but may occasionally occur following trauma or cerebro-vascular disease. It is grossly disabling and unfortunately intractable, although occasional cases improve on high dosage Isoniazid treatment (with pyridoxine supplements) for reasons that are obscure. Doses of Isoniazid up to 900 mg daily may be necessary.

Choreo-athetosis

Abnormal movements which are jerky and non-repetitive may be unilateral or bilateral. When they involve the periphery they are described as "choreo-athetotic" whereas when proximal joints are involved "hemiballismus" or "ballism" may be used.

Choreo-athetosis is seen in a small group of well-defined disorders such as Huntington's chorea, tardive dyskinesia where the face and mouth are mainly involved, and levodopa-treated Parkinson's disease (see Chap. 8). It also occurs sporadically in the elderly when it is usually attributed to non-specific degenerative brain disease. Occasionally chorea results from occult thyrotoxicosis, polycythaemia or systemic lupus erythematosus. Hemiballismus is characteristic of infarction of the subthalamic nucleus. For some reason it is more common in diabetics. The gross flinging uncontrolled limb movements are distressing and exhausting to the patient. It is important to suppress these movements because they may lead to dangerous or even fatal complications before the expected natural recovery can occur. Thus hemiballismus usually substantially (but incompletely) remits within three to four months. In most patients the movements can be suppressed by tetrabenazine. The dose may need to be taken up to levels of 25 mg or even 50 mg three or four times a day. Sedation, depression and parkinsonism are often seen as side effects of this drug. Thiopropazate may be used with success in some cases. Occasionally stereo-tactic surgical thalamotomy has to be resorted to in order to relieve the movement.

The other common disorders causing involuntary movements are discussed in Chapter 8 since they rarely involve the upper limb. But occasionally focal epileptic phenomena may cause diagnostic difficulties when episodic jerking of the arm heralds the development of tumour or infarct in the motor cortex or deep grey matter. The focal partial epilepsies should be treated with carbamazepine or phenytoin in adequate dosage but they may be relatively resistant to anticonvulsant treatment.

Dystonia

A generalised dystonia rarely presents in old age and the only focal dystonia that is seen not uncommonly in the elderly is "writer's cramp".

Writer's cramp used to be considered a "functional" disorder with major psychological overtones. It is now accepted as an organic condition, although patients tend to have personality traits of meticulousness and obsessionality.

Writer's cramp (and the other occupational cramps) more often present in middle life when there are pressures at work to write fast and neatly. The act of writing, and only the act of writing, becomes interrupted and slowed by abnormal posture and tonic muscular contraction. The clues to the diagnosis are to note that the symptoms of disability in the arm are only present when the patient is writing: and on examination there are no abnormal physical signs until the patient attempts to write.

Treatment is nearly always unsatisfactory. The patient must be persuaded to minimise the amount of writing done by using a typewriter, or must learn to write with the left hand, if right-handed.

Dyspraxia

An important but poorly recognised cause of loss of use in the arms is commonly seen but rarely diagnosed in the elderly. Like dyspraxia of gait, dyspraxia for hand movement is a serious disability in old age. The patient, while alert and co-operative, is "fumbly" and "tremulous" so that as soon as she attempts to use her hands to grasp a fork or to attempt to take spectacles from their case the movement is clumsy and interrupted by irregular tremor. Dyspraxia in the hands is less common than dyspraxia of gait. It is usually bilateral and associated with positive grasp and palmo-mental reflexes and generally indicates widespread arteriosclerotic changes in the brain. However, its acute or subacute onset may herald the development of a subdural haematoma, a frontal lesion or a systemic disorder such as cardiac failure or occult infection. Although it may give rise to the suspicion of a parkinsonian syndrome this disorder does not respond to the drugs for parkinsonism. Occupational therapy and re-training techniques may be helpful.

11 Neurological Presentations of General Medical Disorders

Many general medical conditions have neurological complications in the elderly. Neurological symptoms may predominate so that it is commonplace for stroke, epilepsy or other neurological disorder to provide the presenting symptom of underlying disease. In most diseases of the nervous system, therefore, the question should be asked "is this a primary disorder of the nervous system or is it secondary to some other general medical disease?"

Diabetes Mellitus

Most elderly patients with diabetes have the late onset or "maturity" type which pursues an insidious course. The neurological complications of diabetes are common in this group. Patients with peripheral or cerebral vascular disease, neuropathies and visual problems may all have diabetes as a contributory or causative disorder.

Strokes
Diabetes should be considered as a factor in any patient developing a stroke. Although the diagnosis of diabetes is unlikely to influence the risk of further stroke, detection and control of the diabetes may prevent other complications which could adversely affect prognosis. The stroke victim who is also diabetic may, in the context of the acute phase of the stroke, develop keto-acidosis and require insulin therapy. The risk of infection, particularly in the respiratory and urinary tracts, is likely to be greater in stroke patients who are diabetic. And good diabetic control and monitoring may prevent or lessen the impact of, for example, visual deterioration, peripheral neuropathy, neuropathic ulceration, and autonomic neuropathy with postural hypotension.

Peripheral Nerve Damage
Entrapment neuropathies (such as common peroneal nerve palsy or radial palsy) and mononeuropathies – either solitary or multiple – are commonly

associated with, or due to, diabetes mellitus. Neuropathy involving the median nerve (carpal tunnel syndrome) or ulnar nerve, or cervical or lumbar radiculopathy may reflect increased susceptibility of peripheral nerves to pressure or ischaemia.

Peripheral Neuropathy

Many elderly patients with diabetes have what in younger patients would be taken as evidence of a mild, often asymptomatic, peripheral neuropathy, with diminished vibration sense below the knees and absent ankle jerks. As discussed in Chapter 1, many elderly patients without diabetes exhibit these neurological changes and in the elderly diabetic it is difficult to assess, in the absence of other evidence of peripheral nerve involvement, whether these particular signs reflect diabetic neuropathy or not. When the patient complains of sensory abnormalities in the feet it is more likely that a significant neuropathy exists. Some elderly diabetics have marked subjective and objective evidence of neuropathy: symptoms include paraesthesiae, numbness, pain or burning sensations in the legs and feet, and cramps. Examination may reveal objective sensory loss, including all modalities, together with gait ataxia due to abnormalities in joint position sense. In some elderly diabetics, however, objective signs may be minimal or absent when the patient subjectively feels marked pain or paraesthesiae. In other patients subjective features are not prominent but neurological examination reveals conspicuous loss of cutaneous sensory modalities and reflexes: the classical "glove and stocking" anaesthesia may be present but, as with the other features of diabetic peripheral neuropathy, is usually more prominent in the legs than in the arms. Rarely, patients are seen with neuropathic joints due to long-standing or, occasionally, previously undiagnosed diabetes.

Diabetic Amyotrophy

This occurs particularly in elderly diabetics and is characterised by subacute asymmetrical weakness and wasting, often accompanied by pain, affecting the quadriceps muscles. Some patients may complain of back pain as part of the condition. The urethral and anal sphincters may also be involved, leading to incontinence. Diabetic amyotrophy is probably due to vascular changes in the lumbosacral plexus or femoral nerve. Sensory loss is rarely seen in this condition. The symptoms generally resolve slowly over the course of many months but may recur on the previously unaffected side. The pain may be severe and difficult to control, even with regular analgesia.

Autonomic Neuropathy

The common modes of presentation of this complication in elderly diabetics are postural hypotension and diarrhoea. Postural hypotension is often found in the course of investigations for falls and may be the first indication that the patient may be diabetic. Diarrhoea due to autonomic neuropathy may be suspected when other more common causes of diarrhoea and faecal incontinence have been excluded (see Chap.7). In some patients the characteristic explosive nocturnal or early morning diarrhoea occurs but in others diarrhoea of variable severity may occur at any time of day. Hypothermia due to autonomic neuropathy may also lead to a diagnosis of diabetes. Other manifestations of autonomic dysfunction such as diminished sweating and impotence in males are not usually complained of spontaneously. The latter may be assumed by a previously sexually active elderly man to be a manifestation of ageing, to be accepted, therefore, as "normal" and is hence not mentioned unless specific questions are asked. Involvement of the autonomic nerve supply to the bladder may lead to frequency, nocturia and incontinence, each of which may be attributed to other causes of unstable bladder in the elderly, to prostatism in males and to normal ageing by the individual patient and her family. Irregularity of the pupils, miosis and diminished or absent reaction to light may mimic the Argyll–Robertson pupil and with absent ankle jerks and sensory signs has been referred to as "pseudo tabes".

Visual Disorders
In addition to the pupillary changes, other ocular manifestations of diabetes are commonly found in the elderly. Retinopathy should be specifically sought and regular ophthalmic examinations are indicated in elderly patients whose general health and hence life expectancy is good. Cataracts which occur in elderly diabetics are usually indistinguishable from those occuring in non-diabetic individuals. Epidemiological studies indicate, however, that diabetics are prone to develop cataracts at a younger age than non-diabetics and hence may require extraction at a correspondingly younger age.

Hypoglycaemia

The elderly patient with hypoglycaemia may show the familiar features of this condition – sweating, pallor, palpitations, anxiety and mental disturbance. The last may take several forms; the patient may be aggressive, forgetful, drowsy, apparently withdrawn and depressed or may exhibit clouding of consciousness or frank coma. Some patients present with fits, resulting in a misdiagnosis of epilepsy.

Hypoglycaemia in an elderly patient is nearly always due to antidiabetic medication. Any patient presenting with altered consciousness, if known to be diabetic, should be suspected of being hypoglycaemic: the condition is easily treated but if it remains untreated may prove disastrous, resulting in permanent brain damage with cognitive impairment and sometimes focal pyramidal tract signs. Particular diagnostic problems may occur in patients in whom the hypoglycaemia occurs at night: this should be suspected in patients who become uncharacteristically muddled or aggressive in the night, who suffer unexpected nocturnal incontinence, who develop nocturnal fits or who have bad dreams.

Intercurrent illness with loss of appetite or reduced clearance of hypoglycaemic agent may provoke hypoglycaemia. Even mild cognitive changes in the elderly may lead to confusion over dosage, with the resulting hypoglycaemia compounding the problem. Careful supervision of the elderly diabetic must be the rule especially when the patient is forgetful, has poor vision or has any intercurrent illness.

Case 11.1
An 80-year-old female fell at home and was admitted to hospital as an emergency. She was very drowsy but the cause of this was not immediately clear. When her family came to the hospital they informed the staff that the patient was diabetic and took tolbutamide. Blood sugar estimation showed her to be severly hypo-glycaemic and intravenous injection of 50g of glucose resulted in her rapid restoration to full consciousness. Within 2 hours she relapsed into coma from which she was again aroused by intravenous glucose. Over the next few hours this happened on several occasions. Further questioning of her family revealed that about 3 days prior to her fall, as a result of poor eyesight due to diabetic retinopathy, she had mistaken an unlabelled bottle of automobile antifreeze mixture to be a bottle of lemon juice and had consumed a quantity of the sweet-tasting liquid. Urea and electrolyte estimation showed her to have a marked degree of renal failure which had not been present at a previous admission. Blood tolbutamide levels were extremely high. Peritoneal dialysis and repeated intra-venous infusions of glucose over the next few days led to improvement in her renal function, and to her being maintained in a fully conscious state. The renal damage due to antifreeze had led to retention of tolbutamide and consequent hypo-glycaemia. She recovered fully and her diabetes was successfully controlled on the previous dose of tolbutamide.

Other rarer causes of hypoglycaemia may be found in the elderly. It is occasionally seen in patients who have not eaten for a prolonged period. Even rarer are insulin-secreting tumours of the pancreas, or ectopic production of insulin by other tumours.

Thyroid Disease

Myxoedema
Many of the clinical features of hypothyroidism mimic those of ageing. Thus with age the voice deepens, motor activity and responsiveness become slower in the majority of individuals and, particularly in more obese patients, the coarse-ning of features with age produces facies that are easily mistaken for those of myxoedema. Myxoedema in younger individuals may lead to tiredness, leth-argy, muscle aching, weakness and tingling of the hands; many of these symp-toms are, however, common in the elderly and may arise for a variety of reasons. The diagnosis of hypothyroidism may, therefore, be easy to overlook and several neurological disorders may be caused by this condition.

A diagnostic neurological sign of myxoedema is the myotonic tendon reflex which contracts slowly and shows a slow relaxation phase. Many elderly patients, however, have apparently slowed tendon reflex relaxation especially in the ankle jerk and deciding whether the response is abnormal may be difficult.

Carpal tunnel syndrome may be associated with myxoedema and treatment of the hypothyroidism may completely and permanently relieve the symptoms of median nerve entrapment.

Hypothermia with confusion and drowsiness may be the first indication that a patient has myxoedema. The hypothermia arises as a result of diminished heat production associated with the decrease in metabolic rate found in such patients. The patient is particularly vulnerable to cold weather. The failure of thermoregulation may be exacerbated if the patient is ill from another cause (for example a chest infection) as a result of which she fails to eat. Lack of food is thought to impair thermoregulation by suppressing both heat production and conservation. Hypothermia, by definition, is present when the patient's core temperature (taken rectally) is below 35 °C. Any acutely ill elderly patient should be suspected of being at risk of hypothermia and it is important to detect the condition since low body temperature is associated with increased mortality in its own right. If hypothermia is severe the patient may be comatose and the body temperature of any drowsy or unconscious patient should be measured. In these profoundly hypothermic patients it is important not to be deceived by an elevated blood glucose and metabolic acidosis into diagnosing diabetic keto-acidosis. Hyperglycaemia results from insulin resistance as a result of the hypothermia and leads to diminished peripheral utilisation of glucose. The acidosis arises from the accumulation of lactic acid as the enzymes responsible for oxidative phosphorylation are affected by the drop in body temperature. Most patients with these metabolic problems associated with hypothermia are not diabetic and premature use of insulin may result in severe hypoglycaemia as the warming tissues again become responsive to insulin. The metabolic abnormalities usually resolve spontaneously with warming of the patient.

Deafness is very common in the elderly and deafness due to compression of the auditory nerve within the petrous temporal bone due to myxoedema may only become apparent when, after treatment with thyroxine, the severity of deafness diminishes.

Myxoedema as a "reversible" cause of dementia ("myxoedema madness") has been discussed for many years. There appears to be a group of patients with mild impairment of mental function who, with thyroxine, become normal. There is considerable doubt, however, whether these patients really have a true dementia with cognitive impairment; many of the reports of such patients are not validated by use of strict diagnostic criteria for dementia. Other research indicates that myxoedematous patients who are truly demented do not improve with thyroxine: it may well be that patients with mental impairment who do improve with the drug are suffering from mental slowing rather than dementia. That prolonged untreated myxoedema may predispose to multi-infarct dementia is generally accepted and for this reason treatment of myxoedema in the elderly is a priority.

Thyrotoxicosis

The classical features of thyrotoxicosis may be absent in the elderly, or features such as mental change, muscle weakness, tremor and tissue wasting may be attributed to the ageing process, or may be thought to be due to other diseases of old age. The disease may present as an embolic stroke due to thyrotoxic atrial fibrillation or as "funny turns" due to transient cerebral ischaemia. The detection and treatment of thyrotoxicosis and cardioversion to normal rhythm of such patients may be important in preventing further, possibly more serious, cerebral damage.

Occasional patients present with a thyrotoxic myopathy characterised by limb girdle weakness, most noticeable in the pelvic girdle where it affects gait, sometimes with associated muscular fasciculation and diminished tendon reflexes.

In the so-called "apathetic thyrotoxicosis" the patient is listless, slow and lethargic so that a clinical diagnosis of myxoedema may be made despite obvious weight loss. The misdiagnosis of myxoedema is reinforced by the presence of blepharoptosis, which occurs in some patients with apathetic thyrotoxicosis. Patients with this condition may also have muscle wasting or limb girdle myopathy particularly evident in the pelvic girdle.

Disorders of Water and Mineral Metabolism

Disorders of water and mineral metabolism are common in the elderly and mainly reflect changes in renal function which occur in old age, together with the effects of drugs – particularly diuretics – to which the elderly are exposed. The maintenance of normal composition of the extracellular fluid (ECF) is essential to normal cellular function, especially to the electrochemical reactions involved in nerve conduction and muscular contraction. It is therefore to be expected that alterations in the composition of the ECF will result in disturbances of mental function, peripheral nerve conduction and muscle strength.

Water Intoxication
Water intoxication may occur as a result of excessive intravenous fluid therapy, the aged kidney being unable to cope with an increased water load. The condition is also associated with inappropriate secretion of antidiuretic hormone (ADH) which can arise as a result of ectopic production of ADH, most commonly by carcinoma of the bronchus, or in patients with subacute brain diseases (such as meningitis, encephalitis or intoxications) and in some patients with chest infections. There is a severe hyponatraemia but with no evidence of volume depletion or salt loss. The plasma osmolality is lowered and the patient passes an inappropriately concentrated urine. The patient may exhibit muscle weakness or twitching, and slow and diminished tendon jerks. In severe cases the patient may become drowsy or even comatose, and have fits. A rare but potentially recoverable complication of this condition is central pontine myelinolysis causing coma and tetraplegia.

Water Depletion
Water depletion often occurs in sick elderly patients and reflects diminished fluid intake in the presence of decreased renal tubular reabsorption of water.

The patient is usually hypernatraemic. Excess use of diuretics may also lead to water depletion but in this case the patient may be hyponatraemic. Mental changes include increasing confusion, delirium and altered consciousness. Patients with mental change associated with hypernatraemia have sometimes been described as suffering with "hypernatraemic psychosis" and, as a result, have been referred primarily to psychiatric services with gross behavioural disturbance.

Sodium Depletion

Sodium depletion can occur as a result of excessive loss of sodium from disease (diarrhoea, diabetic keto-acidosis, pyrexia with excessive sweating), from diuretic therapy and, rarely in the elderly, Addison's disease. The patient may exhibit lassitude, apathy, muscle weakness and cramps, and have mental changes, in particular disorientation in time and space, clouding of consciousness, delusions and visual hallucinations.

Potassium Depletion

The commonest cause of potassium depletion in the elderly is diuretic therapy, particularly with thiazide diuretics. Specific mental and neurological sequelae include depression, apathy, paranoid states and muscle weakness.

Hyperkalaemia

Hyperkalaemia may occur as a result of renal failure and even in relatively mild renal failure may be precipitated by use of potassium-sparing diuretics. The patient may become lethargic and confused and in severe cases may have flaccid paralysis of the muscles.

Magnesium Depletion

Magnesium is contained in a wide variety of foods and dietary deficiency of magnesium does not generally occur in the absence of marked protein calorie malnutrition. Magnesium depletion may be more common in the elderly than is generally appreciated and results mainly from excess renal loss of magnesium due to diuretic therapy. Severe diarrhoeal illnesses may also lead to magnesium depletion. Increased loss of magnesium from the kidney occurs in excessive alcohol ingestion both as a result of a direct action of alcohol on the renal tubule and from secondary hyperaldosteronism found in alcoholics with cirrhosis. The patient may be depressed, irritable and ataxic, have muscle weakness and complain of vertigo. In severe examples carpopedal spasm may be found, together with positive Chvostek's and Trousseau's signs, athetoid movements and convulsions.

Disorders of Calcium Metabolism

The neuropsychiatric effects found in disorders of calcium metabolism are primarily due to the alteration in level of serum calcium rather than to the underlying condition. Transient alterations in serum calcium, both hypocalcaemia and hypercalcaemia, are seen in sick elderly patients: the former is usually mild and resolves spontaneously when the patient recovers from the underlying illness; the latter may be due to salt and water depletion and resolves with rehydration and salt loading. Other patients have persistent changes in the serum calcium and it is in this group that the neuropsychiatric effects are most apparent.

Hypercalcaemia

The common causes of hypercalcaemia in the elderly are listed in Table 11.1. Symptoms include depression, lassitude, constipation, delirium (which may be marked in severe hypercalcaemia), clouding of consciousness, intellectual impairment, and muscle weakness. If the serum calcium is very high the patient may become comatose. All these features resolve as the calcium is restored to the normal range by appropriate therapy.

Hypocalcaemia

The common causes of hypocalcaemia in the elderly are listed in Table 11.1. The characteristic features of positive Chvostek's and Trousseau's sign may be found in severe cases and in some patients carpopedal spasm, generalised convulsions, psychotic behavioural disturbance, stupor, coma and raised intracranial pressure with papilloedema may be observed. Chorea is a rare presentation of hypocalcaemia. In most elderly patients with hypocalcaemia, however, these florid signs are absent, the hypocalcaemia being relatively mild. Prolonged hypocalcaemia as seen in osteomalacia may result in a proximal myopathy particularly obvious in the pelvic girdle, producing a waddling gait. The tendon reflexes are typically increased. Insidious intellectual impairment may also be found in conjunction with hypocalcaemia, correction of the latter often leading to gradual restoration of normal cognition.

Table 11.1. Common disorders of calcium metabolism in the elderly.

Hypercalcaemia
  Malignancy
    Ectopic production of parathormone
    Skeletal metastases
    Haematological disorders (e.g., myeloma, lymphoma)
  Primary hyperparathyroidism
  Artefactual
    venous stasis
    hyperalbuminaemia (dehydration)

Hypocalcaemia
  Osteomalacia
  Chronic renal disease
  Low plasma albumin
    malnutrition or malabsorption
    liver disease
  Acute pancreatitis

Alcohol and Alcoholism

Particular aspects of alcohol-related neurological disease have already been discussed when considering the amnesic states and dementia. Alcohol is an important cause of neurological disability in the elderly. It has replaced syphilis as the great mimic of other conditions and, like venereal disease, the crucial features in the history are typically concealed by the patient and often by her family as well.

Recent studies suggest that over 10% of elderly individuals living in the community may consume quantities of alcohol which would be anticipated to be associated with alcohol-related disease. In geriatric practice the more alcohol ingestion is sought as a factor in acutely-admitted patients the more often it is found. The elderly alcoholic often presents to the geriatrician rather than to the psychogeriatrician with primarily physical problems – falls, immobility and incontinence being common reasons for admission. Any of these presentations should alert the physician to possible alcohol abuse by an elderly patient.

Elderly alcoholics fall roughly into two groups, those who have a long history of alcoholism – graduate alcoholics – and those who take up alcohol late in life often as a result of stress or bereavement or as a social bonding with others, for example other family members who are themselves alcoholic (the alcoholic folie à deux). The graduate alcoholic, being a survivor, is often relatively fit, probably as a reflection of a pattern of drinking which in economic terms has allowed for adequate food intake, the effects of nutritional deficiency thus being absent. The elderly patient in whom heavy drinking is of relatively recent onset may, either as a result of alcoholic gastritis or because she cannot afford to drink and eat, be more likely to suffer nutritional side effects and hepatic damage.

Peripheral Neuropathy
In the early stages alcoholic peripheral neuropathy may produce few physical signs apart from loss of the ankle jerks – a phenomenon common in the elderly anyway. Often, however, the patient complains of sensory disturbance with burning sensations in the feet, numbness, pins and needles and pain. The associated muscle weakness may lead to foot drop and the appearance of a high-stepping gait: the leg muscles show evidence of wasting (though in thin elderly patients this may be difficult to assess) and absent knee and ankle jerks. Cutaneous loss is predominantly peripheral in distribution. The skin may be intensely hyperaesthesic. Alcoholic peripheral neuropathy may be seen in isolation, though in 50% of patients so affected features of, or residual effects from, other alcohol-related neurological syndromes such as Wernicks's encephalopathy and Korsakoff's psychosis are seen. The neuropathy is generally thought to be due to thiamine deficiency, though lack of other B-group vitamins cannot be ruled out. Treatment with vitamin supplementation is usually associated with some degree of recovery though the patient may suffer with residual effects to a varying degree.

Cerebellar Degeneration

Cerebellar degeneration usually develops over the course of several weeks or months and then remains static for a number of years. The main features are an ataxia of stance and of gait, other features of cerebellar disorder often being absent. The cause is thought to be nutritional rather than a direct toxic effect of the alcohol.

Wernicke's Encephalopathy

Wernicke's encephalopathy is the acute neuropsychiatric reaction to deficiency of thiamine, and alcoholism is the commonest cause of this condition in western society. The classical presentation is the sudden onset of confusion, ataxia and ophthalmoplegia, though not all these features are necessarily seen together. The mental changes are often referred to as "quiet global confusion" with disorientation in space and time, apathy and cognitive impairment: some patients show evidence of mild delirium, with perceptual distortions and hallucinations going on to drowsiness or even coma. Confused patients are often evasive and cover up their mental deficits with facile conversation and, perhaps more typically, confabulation. The ataxia observed in patients with Wernicke's encephalopathy may vary from a mild abnormality in the heel-toe walking test to a total inability to stand; intention tremor is relatively rare. The ocular abnormalities are seen in the majority of patients with this condition. The commonest are nystagmus, sixth cranial nerve palsies and conjugate gaze paralysis. The pupillary reactions may be sluggish but this finding is so common in the elderly that it is very difficult to be certain when the finding represents significant underlying pathology. The ocular abnormalities respond very rapidly to treatment or to feeding with food containing thiamine and unless looked for specifically at the time of the first consultation may be missed.

Wernicke's encephalopathy is an extremely serious condition with a high mortality. Any patient in whom the diagnosis is possible should have blood taken for thiamine estimation and immediate intravenous thiamine should be administered.

Korsakoff's Psychosis

It is likely that Korsakoff's psychosis is another facet of thiamine deficiency and represents a more extreme and chronic reaction than Wernicke's encephalopathy. Many patients with Wernicke's encephalopathy have severe persistent memory impairment characteristic of Korsakoff's psychosis, with otherwise well-preserved cognitive function. Thus psychometric tests of memory will be abnormal but those of standard intelligence will be within the normal range.

Alcoholic Dementia

The existence of alcoholic dementia remains somewhat controversial. In a patient who drinks heavily and for a prolonged period, chronic inebriation may lead to global impairment of cognition. With abstinence this cognitive deficit may take many months to improve and, by virtue of its apparent chronicity may be misdiagnosed as a dementing process. It is likely that excessive alcohol intake increases the risk of vascular disease and, as a result of this, arteriosclerotic dementia may be more common in alcoholics and hence be described as "alcoholic dementia". In the elderly, senile dementia of the Alzheimer type also becomes more common and it is, therefore, likely that in elderly alcoholics who coincidentally have senile dementia the latter will again be labelled as "alcoholic dementia". There is, however, an increasing body of literature suggesting that chronic alcoholic excess causes a specific dementia syndrome.

Alcohol Withdrawal

This may be undertaken as a therapeutic measure but may occur as a result of unintentional cessation of alcohol ingestion when, for example, the patient is admitted to hospital for another cause. Alcohol withdrawal should always be considered as the cause when an unexplained confusional state develops in an elderly patient who was admitted to hospital apparently mentally normal several days earlier. Milder forms of withdrawal states include features such as tremor, weakness, nausea and irritability. In more severe forms predominantly visual hallucinations may be present, together with tinnitus, abnormal visual phenomena (blurrring, flashes of light and spots in the visual field) and convulsions in patients with several years of addiction.

Case 11.2

An 82-year-old female, normally resident in a block of wardened flatlets, was admitted from the Accident and Emergency Department following a fall at home. She was found to be very unsteady on her feet and considered to be unsafe to return home without further investigation and rehabilitation. When first admitted to the ward she appeared to be quite cheerful and well orientated in time and space. Two days afterwards she was noticed to have become rather irritable in her manner, had a tremor of her hands and was nauseated. She also complained of seeing young girls on the ward who were pestering her. Blood tests showed her to have a macrocytosis and elevation of serum alkaline phosphatase and γ-glutamyl transferase. These findings led to specific questioning of the warden of the flatlets and the patient's home help about possible alcohol ingestion by the patient. It transpired that she had been drinking a bottle of whisky and numbers of cans of lager a week for several years following the death of her husband. The fall which had brought her to the hospital was the most recent and most severe of a series that had started about a year prior to admission. Over the following 10 days her agitation and visual hallucinations settled down and she became safely mobile with a walking stick. With the patient's agreement the supplier of her alcohol (another well-meaning elderly resident in the same block of flats) stopped bringing in the patient's "supplies" and no further falls or episodes of agitation or visual hallucinosis occurred in the following year.

Delirium Tremens

Delirium tremens represents the most severe form of alcohol withdrawal. The onset is often at night and may be very sudden. The patient is restless, unable to sleep and fearful. Sleep may be disturbed by vivid nightmares, the patient waking in a panic. As the reaction progresses the patient becomes increasingly anxious, and restless. Dehydration may be a prominent feature and the patient rapidly reaches a point of total physical exhaustion. There is evidence of intense autonomic arousal with profuse sweating, pallor, a rapid small volume pulse and sometimes a mild.pyrexia. The patient experiences a profusion of hallucinations and illusions, often changing rapidly in form, but vivid and producing intense emotional response. The patient is usually frightened by the hallucinations, but sometimes inappropriate gaiety is seen, interspersed with periods of apprehension. The patient exhibits a general lack of awareness of her surroundings. Over the course of about 3 days the patient lapses into sleep and on waking feels fully recovered but exhausted. Death may occur due to intercurrent infection (particularly of the respiratory tract) cardiovascular collapse, hyperthermia or self injury.

The exact cause of alcohol withdrawal syndromes is not known. Magnesium deficiency is common in heavy drinkers due both to a direct toxic effect of alcohol on renal tubular reabsorption of magnesium and to hyperaldosteronism secondary to alcoholic cirrhosis. This magnesium deficiency has been proposed as a cause of withdrawal symptoms, but the evidence for this remains uncertain. Magnesium repletion therapy in this situation will, however, prevent some of the other effects of magnesium depletion, including cardiac dysrrhythmias, muscle weakness, hypokalaemia and hypocalcaemia and should, therefore, be undertaken.

Nutritional and other Vitamin Deficiencies

Pellagra
Pellagra may manifest as an acute organic brain reaction with disorientation and memory loss. The patient may also be depressed and exhibit a paranoid state with hallucinosis and delusions. The classical triad of "dermatitis, diarrhoea and dementia" (the last being a misnomer) may be misinterpreted in the elderly: many elderly patients have rashes; many, particularly those with impaction of faeces, have diarrhoea; and many have mental changes due to a variety of causes. Nicotinic acid deficiency is probably the primary cause of the condition and occurs in elderly individuals who are living in circumstances of extreme neglect. Treatment with nicotinic acid usually results in rapid reversal of the neuropsychiatric features of the condition.

Subacute Combined Degeneration of the Cord
The neuropathy due to deficiency of vitamin B_{12} affects not only the spinal cord but also the peripheral nerves and higher mental function. The condition may occur without any anaemia or other haematological changes in the blood film or bone marrow. In elderly patients the features of the disease (subjective complaints of tingling and numbness of the extremities, and pain; weakness, ataxia, diminution of sensibility to light touch, pin-prick, heat and cold, loss of joint-position sensation, diminished tendon reflexes in the lower limb and extensor plantar response) may not be noticed by the patient, may be difficult to elicit and

may be interpreted as being due to other causes. The condition is so treatable that any patient with evidence of peripheral sensory abnormality, or progressive alteration in gait should have her serum vitamin B_{12} measured. The issue of dementia resulting from vitamin B_{12} deficiency is discussed in Chapter 3.

Folic Acid Deficiency
There is some evidence that this condition may be associated with damage to the spinal cord and peripheral neuropathy. Such manifestations of folic acid deficiency, which is a relatively common condition, seem to be rare and hence there remains some doubt as to whether the primary cause of the neurological changes is folic acid deficiency. But some patients with malabsorption syndromes or nutritional deficiency develop sensory symptoms which appear to be relieved by a course of treatment with folic acid.

Neuropsychiatric Manifestations of Malignant Disease

The general incidence of malignant disease increases with age and it is, therefore, not surprising that neuropsychiatric manifestations of malignant disease are not uncommonly seen in the very elderly. The syndromes observed fall into two categories; firstly, those in which neurological change is observed when neither the primary nor secondary growths are anatomically sited in a position which will explain the neurological abnormality (the so-called "non-metastatic" manifestation) and, secondly, those in which the primary or secondary growths cause the neurological change by their physical presence and anatomical location.

Non-metastatic Neurological Manifestations
The list of syndromes reported so far includes motor or sensory peripheral neuropathy, cerebellar degeneration, spinal cord degeneration, dementia, encephalomyelitis, meningitis, myopathy, myositis and myasthenia. In elderly patients it is easy to attribute signs from one of the above conditions to cerebro-vascular disease. In the early stages of the condition, one of the most useful diagnostic features is the subacute onset and steady progression of the non-metastatic syndromes as opposed to the sudden onset and stepwise progression found in cerebro-vascular disease. Such clinical distinctions are not always possible, however, and underlying malignancy should always be considered in any patient who has an atypical presentation of a neurological abnormality. The carcinomas most commonly producing neurological syndromes are, in order of frequency, bronchus, stomach and ovary.

Local Neurological Manifestations
Cerebral metastases may produce focal signs, behavioural disturbance, dysphasias and dyspraxias according to their situation and may also lead to

convulsions. Again the problem diagnostically is in distinguishing the more common cerebro-vascular disease from malignancy. The evolution of the condition – gradual onset and progression in the malignant syndromes – may be the most useful feature, but typical stroke syndrome can occur when sudden haemorrhage into or infarction of a tumour occurs. The subsequent clinical progression may suggest malignancy; for example, if after an apparent stroke the patient continues to "go downhill" without evidence of concurrent infection or heart failure, or shows a progressive neurological abnormality.

Peripheral nerve compression syndromes are also seen; that due to a Pancoast tumour from apical carcinoma of the bronchus is perhaps the commonest example. Here intractible pain in the arm is associated with a Horner's syndrome and ipsilateral T1 root signs with wasting of the hand and sensory loss over the inside of the elbow.

Herpes Zoster

Shingles

Shingles is most commonly seen in patients over the age of 50 years and continues to increase in incidence into late life. A detailed description of the disease and its pathophysiology is inappropriate to the present text and mention has already been made in the section on facial pain. But there are several points about the condition in the elderly which need to be emphasised. Many elderly patients will present with pain before the rash appears and recognition of the condition at this stage offers the best prospect of early treatment and hence of preventing post-herpetic neuralgia. At this stage, local therapy with idoxuridine and systemic therapy with acyclovir may lead to rapid resolution of the skin lesions and a low incidence of post-herpetic neuralgia. Oral acyclovir accelerates recovery from the skin rash but does not seem to affect the incidence of post-herpetic neuralgia. However steroids (prednisolone 40mg daily reducing over 2 weeks) reduces the incidence of intractible pain from neuralgia and does not seem to carry excess risk of viraemia.

The treatment of post-herpetic neuralgia is extremely difficult. Opiate analgesics are not appropriate, but simple analgesics seldom affect the pain significantly. Antidepressant drugs combined with anticonvulsants such as valproate or carbamezepine seem to be the most effective form of therapy.

Motor radiculopathy or sphincter disturbance with incontinence are rare complications of herpes zoster. Recovery is slow and usually incomplete.

Herpes Encephalomyelitis

The neurological complications of zoster become increasingly rare as the central nervous system is ascended. Necrotising myelitis, encephalitis and even meningitis have been reported. The prognosis has been transformed by the introduction of treatment with acyclovir.

Myeloma and the Dysproteinaemias

Plasma hyperviscosity in myeloma and the dysproteinaemias may predispose to stroke. Rarely, a solitary plasmacytoma may act as a compressive lesion to the spinal cord, orbit or even within the cranium. But the most important neurological presentation with myeloma or the dysproteinaemias is a neuropathy. Usually there is a generalised peripheral sensorimotor neuropathy with peripheral demyelination. Occasionally there may be a multiple mono-neuropathic presentation. The neurological symptoms and signs not uncommonly far precede the other manifestations of the myeloma.

Treatment of the myeloma may give useful remission of symptoms and some patients respond well to treatment with steroids or ACTH.

Drugs

Tardive (Orofacial) Dyskinesia

These abnormal involuntary movements affecting the face and sometimes the trunk and limbs occur in patients who have been treated with neuroleptic medication. The phenothiazines are mainly responsible (whether as psychiatric treatment, as anti-emetics, or as commonly – and inappropriately – given for the treatment of postural instability or non-specific "giddiness"). But butyrophenones may also provoke the continuous choreo-athetoid movements. Akathisia, a pathological restlessness, may also be seen. Withdrawal of the drug seldom leads to reduction of the movements which may, in fact, increase. Some patients taking phenothiazines show no evidence of dyskinesia but withdrawal of the drug may lead to the appearance of abnormal movements.

Tardive dyskinesia increases in incidence with age and is much more common in patients with chronic schizophrenic illness. By contrast, acute dystonic reactions from phenothiazines are very rare in the elderly.

Up to 50% of cases of tardive dyskinesia recover within 3 years of withdrawing the drug that provoked the disorder. In severe cases suppression of the movements may be achieved with tetrabenazine, but treatment is in general unsatisfactory. However, the severity of the movements is usually perceived more by the family or the physician than by the patient who may be able to ignore the movements to a remarkable degree.

Drug-induced Neuropathy

Drug-induced neuropathy is almost always due to a drug-induced axonal degeneration within the affected nerves. A number of drugs have been reported as producing polyneuropathies (see Table 11.2). Nitrofurantoin may cause a mixed motor and sensory neuropathy in patients who develop excessively high blood levels as a result of failure of excretion secondary to renal impairment: the elderly by virtue of the prevalence of diminished renal function are particularly

Table 11.2. Drugs producing peripheral neuropathy

Nitrofurantoin
Isoniazid
Vincristine (also an autonomic neuropathy)
Perhexiline maleate
Hydralizine (at high doses)
Amioderone
Penicillamine
Imipramine
Anticonvulsants (e.g., phenytoin)
Metronidazole
Gold therapy

at risk. Isoniazid can also lead to a motor and sensory neuropathy and this is more likely to occur in patients who are slow acetylators of the drug. This complication can be prevented by concurrent prescription of pyridoxine.

Great caution must be exercised in the elderly when prescribing these drugs and where there is any renal impairment drug levels should be monitored.

References and Further Reading

References

Dujovny M, Charbel F, Berman SK, Diaz FG, Malik G, Ausman JI (1987) Geriatric neurosurgery. Surg Neurol 29: 10–16

Folstein MF et al. (1975) *"Mini-mental state" a practical method of grading the cognitive state of patients for the clinician.* J Psychiatr Res 12: 189–198

Hachinski VC et al. (1975) *Cerebral blood flow in dementia.* Arch Neurol 32: 632–637

Mulley GP (ed) (1989) *Aids and appliances* British Medical Journal, London.

Norton D, Maclaren R, Exton-Smith AN (1962) *An investigation of geriatric nursing problems in hospital.* Centre for Policy on Ageing, London

Qureshi K, Hodkinson MH (1974) Evaluation of a ten question mental test in the institutionalised elderly. Age Ageing 3: 152–157

Further Reading

Albert ML (ed) (1984) *Clinical neurology of ageing.* Oxford University Press, New York

Brocklehurst JC (ed) (1985) *Textbook of geriatric medicine and gerontology*, Churchill Livingstone, Edinburgh.

Caird FI (ed) (1982) *Neurological disorders in the elderly*, J.Wright, Bristol

Hildick Smith M (ed) (1985) *Neurological problems in the elderly*, Bailliere Tindall, London

Lishman WA (1987) *Organic psychiatry: the psychological consequences of cerebral disorders*, Blackwell Scientific Publications, Oxford

Mathews WB (1975) *Practical neurology*, Blackwell Scientific Publications, Oxford

Pathy MSJ (ed) (1985) *Principles and practice of geriatric medicine*, Wiley, Chichester

Tallis RC (ed) (1989) *The clinical neurology of old age*, Wiley, Chichester

Toghill PJ (ed) (1989) *Physical signs in clinical medicine*, Edward Arnold, London

Vinken PJ, Bruyn GW, Klawans HL (eds) *Handbook of clinical neurology,* Elsevier, Amsterdam (A multivolume text published over a number of years).

Warlow C (1985) *Strokes*, MTP, Lancaster

Wilkinson IMS (1988) *Essential neurology*, Blackwell Scientific Publications, Oxford.

Subject Index

Abbreviated Mental Test   30
Abnormal movement disorders   98–99,
    123–125
Absent-mindedness   25
Aids and appliances   8, 52, 119
Akathisia   93
Alcohol and alcoholism   85, 135–138
Alcohol withdrawal   137
Alcoholic cirrhosis   138
Alcoholic dementia   35, 136–137
Alcoholic neuropathy   48
Alzheimer's disease   36–37, 50, 95, 111
    type 1 (AD1)   36
    type 2 (AD2)   36
Amantadine   97
Amaurosis fugax   68
Amnesic states   108–111
Aneurysms   18, 23, 59–60
Anticholinergic agents   83, 97–99
Antidiuretic hormone (ADH)   132
Antihypertensive agents   8
Angiography   22–23
Apathetic thyrotoxicosis   132
Appliances   8, 52, 119
Argyll–Robertson pupil   129
Arm
    disturbance of function in   113
    neuropathic weakness of   114–119
    see also Upper limb
Arthritis   57, 113, 120
Arthropathic weakness   118
Atypical facial pain   see facial pain
Autonomic function disturbances   93–94
Autonomic neuropathy   128, 129

Babcock sentence   29
Baclofen in dystonic dysarthria   99
Balance disorders   43, 45
Ballism   123–124

Basal meningiomas   18, 50
Benedikt's syndrome   74
Bell's palsy   56
Benign intracranial hypertension   17
Benign positional vertigo   45–46
Benzhexol   98–99
Binswanger's encephalopathy   33, 38, 39, 50
Bladder   77–83
    disturbance in parkinsonism   90, 93
    effect of ageing   79
    normal control   78
Blood pressure   8, 102, 104, 106, 107, 128
Body temperature   7, 108
Bone pain   58
Bowel function   80, 83–85, 93, 128
Brain abscess   15
Brain injury   17
Brain tumour   53, 61, 117, 120, 121
Brainstem disorders   21, 74, 107
Bromocriptine in Parkinson's disease   97, 98
Brown–Sequard hemicord lesion   122

Calcium metabolism disorders   133–134
Carbamazepine in trigeminal neuralgia   63
Cardiac dysrrhythmias   105
Carotid artery, emboli in   68, 69
Carpal tunnel syndrome   113, 122
Cataract   45, 129
Cauda equina   21, 83
Central pontine myelinolysis   35
Cerebellar degeneration   9, 47, 136
Cerebral tumour   15, 17, 18, 19, 32, 61, 76,
    82, 105, 117
Cerebrospinal fluid (CSF)   15–17
Cervical spondylosis   57, 113, 118, 120
Cervical spondylotic myelopathy   11, 118
Choreo-athetosis   123–124
Chronic subdural haematoma (CSDH) 17,
    18, 60

Cognitive impairment   25–29, 35–42, 92
Coma   19, 101, 108, 129
Computed tomography (CT) scan   15–18,
    51, 53, 105
Confabulation   3, 27, 110
Confusion   9, 25–35, 42, 110
    causes of   32
    examination in   28–30
    history-taking   26–28
    use of term   25
Consciousness disturbance   101–108
    history, examination and investigation
        in   103
Constipation   80, 90, 93, 99
Cord lesions   21, 47, 82–83, 117–119, 121
Cortical sensory defects   121
Costen's syndrome   57
Cough syncope   106
Cranial arteritis   54–56
Crutches palsy   119

Deafness   2–3, 5
Decarboxylase inhibitor in Parkinson's
    disease   97–98
Defaecation control   83–85
Dehydration   9, 137
Delirium   32–36
Delirium tremens   36, 137–138
Dementia   3, 9, 17, 19, 32, 35–40
    Alzheimer type   36–37
    causes of   32
    definitive diagnosis   25
    early stages of   3
    frontal type   40–41
    incorrect diagnosis of   2
    Parkinson's disease and   40, 90, 93, 95–96
    Pseudodementia   27, 41–42
    reversible   39
    subcortical   39–40
    vascular   37–39
Depression 2, 41–42, 49, 61, 93, 98
Dexamethasone   18
Diabetes mellitus   120, 122, 124, 127–129
Diabetic amyotrophy   128
Diffuse Lewy body disease   40, 50, 95–99
Dislocation of the shoulder   119
Dizziness   5, 8, 45–46, 106
Dopamine agonists   50, 51
    in Parkinson's disease   95–98
Double vision   68, 72–75
Drop attacks   106–107
Drowsiness   101, 107–109
Drug-induced neuropathy see Neuropathy
Drugs   4, 28, 34, 141–142
Dysphasia   27, 29, 30, 117
Dyspraxia   27, 124–125
Dysproteinaemias   141

Dystonia   98–99, 124
Dystonic dysarthria   6, 99

Eaton–Lambert syndrome   20, 117
ECG   101, 105
EEG   18–20, 34, 101, 102, 105
EMG   20–21
Encephalitis   27
ENT examination   56
Epilepsy   18, 19, 26, 70, 102–105, 124
ESR   55
Evoked potential recording   21
Examination   1–11

Facial dyskinesia   99, 123
Facial neuralgia   53, 62–65
Facial pain (atypical)   64–65
Faecal incontinence   77, 83–85
    causes of   84
    examination   85
    history-taking   85
Fainting   93, 104, 106
Falls   43–52, 118–119
Fasciculation   10, 20, 115
Folic acid deficiency   139
Footwear   6
Foster–Kennedy syndrome   71
Frontal lobe incontinence   82

Gait disturbance   9, 17, 41, 43–52, 90
Gait dyspraxia   49–52
    causes of   50
    physiology of   51
    treatment of   51–52
Ganglion or root thermocoagulation   63
General examination   5–7
General paralysis of the insane (GPI)   51
Glioma   see Brain tumour
Glossopharyngeal neuralgia   64
Guillain–Barré syndrome   21, 48, 74

Hachinski score   39
Hallucinations   27, 28, 75–76, 110
Head injury   17, 101
Headache   18, 53–62
    causes of   54
    chronic   54
    diagnosis of   53
    extracranial   54–58
    from ENT or dental conditions   56
    intracranial   58–61
    psychogenic   61–62
Hearing aids   3, 5
Hearing loss   5

Hemiballismus 123, 124
Hemicord lesions 122
Hemiparesis 5, 11, 17, 18, 47, 117
Herpes encephalomyelitis 140
Herpes zoster 5, 56, 64, 71, 84, 115, 117, 140
History-taking 2–5
  faecal incontinence 85
  headache 53
  impaired mental function 26–28
  loss of consciousness 103
  loss of use in hand or arm 114
  urinary incontinence 79–80, 90
Horner's syndrome 68, 116, 140
Huntington's chorea 32, 100, 123
Hypercalcaemia 134
Hyperkalaemia 133
Hypertension 8, 68, 107
Hypocalcaemia 134
Hypoglycaemia 102, 129–130
Hypokinesia 90, 91
Hypotension 8, 102, 104, 106, 128
Hypothermia 7, 108

Iatrogenic illness 4
Iceberg phenomenon 6
Idiopathic Bell's palsy see Bell's palsy
Idiopathic blepharospasm 98–99
Incontinence 77–86, 90
  nocturnal 79
  see also Faecal incontinence; Urinary
    incontinence
Indomethacin in postural hypotension 106
Intrinsic lesions of the spinal cord 122
Investigation 13–23
Isoniazid, neuropathy due to 142

Jakob–Creutzfeldt disease 32, 72

Korsakoff's psychosis 35, 109–110, 135, 136

Language see dysphasia
Lateral medulla, lesions of 121
Levodopa in Parkinson's disease 97, 98,
  99, 124
Lumbar puncture 15–17, 22
Lumbo-sacral plexus lesions 83

Magnesium deficiency 133, 138
Magnetic resonance imaging (MRI) 23
Malignant disease 13
  local neurological manifestations 139–140
  neuropsychiatric manifestations 139–140
  non-metastatic neurological
    manifestations 139–140

Malignant meningitis 17
Marchiafava–Bignami disease 35
Median neuropathy 116, 119
Memory assessment 2, 3, 29–31, 108, 109
Memory disturbance 108–111
Memory tests 29–31, 108
Meniérès disease 45
Meningioma 61
Meningitis 16, 27
Mental function
  assessment of 2–3, 28–31, 39, 109
  impairment in 25–26, 35–42, 108–111
Micturition syncope 106
Migraine 58, 69–70
Mineral metabolism disorders 132–134
Mini-mental state examination 31
Motor neurone disease 20, 115, 116, 120
Motor system 46–47
Multi-infarct dementia 10, 37–39, 92, 111
Multi-system atrophy 50, 51, 92
Multiple sclerosis 21
Multiple Sensory Dizziness Syndrome
  (MSDS) 46
Muscle power see Muscle weakness
Muscle tone, upper limb 115–116
Muscle wasting 10, 116
Muscle weakness 47, 48, 116–119
Musculo-skeletal disorders 47–48, 90, 118,
  120
Myasthenia gravis 20, 117
Myasthenic syndrome 20, 117
Myelography 21–22
Myeloma 141
Myopathy 20, 107, 117
Myotonia 20
Myxoedema 2, 130–131

Nerve conduction velocity (NCV) 20–21
Neuralgic amyotrophy 117
Neurological examination 8–11
Neuro-ophthalmological problems 68–75
  examination 67, 68
Neuropathies 48
  drug related 141–142
Nicotinic acid deficiency 35
Nitrofurantoin, neuropathy due to 141–142
Nocturnal behavioural disturbance 34
Normal pressure hydrocephalus 41, 50, 51, 82
Numbness in upper limb 119–122
Nutritional deficiency 35, 138, 139

Occipital neuralgias 57
Onychogryphosis 6
Ophthalmoplegia 17, 72–75

Organic brain syndromes, acute and
        subacute 32–35
    causes of 33
    mechanisms underlying 34
    see also Dementia
Oro-facial-dyskinesia 6, 99, 123
Osteoarthritis 43, 44, 118

Paget's disease 54, 58
Palmo-mental reflex 10, 115
Pancoast tumour 116, 140
Paraplegia 5, 22, 43, 47, 48
Paratonia 115
Parinaud's syndrome 74
Parkinsonism 49, 50, 87–99, 125
    assessment of 88, 94, 97
    autonomic function in 93–94
    classification of 92
    course of 94–95
    diagnosis of 87, 88
    disorders of higher mental function 40, 93,
        95
    examination 90–94
    of known aetiology 92
    presenting symptoms and signs of 88–90
    prevalence of 88
    primary idiopathic 92
    see also Senile Parkinsonism
Parkinson's disease 2, 3, 5, 6, 9, 47, 49–51, 87,
        88, 95–99, 115
    and dementia 40, 90, 93, 95
    clinical features 88–96
    diagnosis of 88
    levodopa-treated 97–99
    management of 96–99
Pellagra 34, 35, 138
Peripheral mononeuropathies 122, 127, 128
    nerve conduction in 20
Peripheral nerve compression syndromes 122,
        140
Peripheral neurectomy 63
Peripheral neuropathy 122, 128, 135
    drugs producing 142
Phenothiazine anti-emetics 46, 92
Pick's disease 41
Pituitary apoplexy 33
Pituitary tumour 33, 61
Plantar reflexes 10
Posterior fossa microvascular
        decompression 64
Post-herpetic neuralgia 64
Post-stroke narcolepsy 107–108
Postural hypotension 8, 93, 104, 106
Postural unsteadiness 43 ,
Posture maintenance 44–48
Potassium depletion 133

Prechiasmal lesions 71–72
Pressure sores 6, 7
Primitive reflexes 10
Progressive supra-nuclear palsy 75, 92, 94
Proprioception abnormality 44–48, 121, 122
Prosopagnosia 76
Pseudo tabes 129
Pseudobulbar palsy 37
Pseudodementia 27, 41–42
Pseudo-Foster–Kennedy syndrome 71
Psychogenic attacks 102
Pyridoxine in isoniazid neuropathy 142

Ramsay–Hunt syndrome 56
Retrobulbar lesions 71–72
Retrochiasmal lesions 72
Rheumatoid arthritis 57, 118
Rigidity 90, 91
Root lesions 83, 122
Rooting reflex 10

Seborrhoea 93
Selegiline in Parkinsonism 97–98
Senile parkinsonism 40, 95–98
    management of 96–98
Sensory examination 119–122
Shingles see Herpes zoster
Sinus pain 56
Skin diseases 6
Snellen chart 6, 67
Sodium depletion 133
Spasmodic torticollis 98
Spectacles 6, 67
Speech abnormalities and assessment see
        dysphasia
Spinal cord lesions 82, 117, 118, 121, 122
Steele–Richardson–Olszewski
        syndrome 39–40, 75, 92, 94
Sticks 119
Stroke 18, 32, 37, 47, 50, 59, 69, 82, 102, 107,
        108, 117, 127
Stupor 19, 32
Subacute combined degeneration of the cord
        48, 138
Subarachnoid haemorrhage 15, 16, 27, 59–60
Subclavian steal syndrome 22
Subcortical arteriosclerotic
        encephalopathy 50
Subdural haematoma see Chronic subdural
        haematoma
Syringomyelia 117, 122

Tardive dyskinesia 123, 141
Temporo-mandibular arthropathy 57

Tendon reflexes   9, 117
Tetrabenazine
   in abnormal involuntary movements   99,
      124
   in tardive dyskinesia   141
Thalamic lesions   121
Thiamine deficiency   136
Thoracic outlet syndromes   116
Thought block   93
Thyroid disease   130–132
Thyrotoxicosis   131–132
Toxic confusional states   35
Transient global amnesia   110–111
Transient ischaemic attack   59, 68, 69, 111
Trauma   17, 117
Traumatic neuropathies   118, 119
Tremor   87, 89–91, 123
Triceps jerks   10, 118
Trigeminal neuralgia   62–64
   surgical treatment of   63–64
Tumours   see Cerebral tumours

Ulcers   6
Ulnar neuropathy   116
Upper limb
   classification of causes for loss of use in   120
   examination   114–122
   history-taking   113, 114
   inspection   115
   loss of use of   113–125
   muscle tone   115–116
   sensory loss in   119–122
   signs of loss of use in   115–119
Upper spinal lesions   82, 117, 118, 122
Urinary incontinence   41, 77–83
   causes of   81–83

examination and investigation   80–81
history-taking   79–80
Urinary tract disease   80

Vascular (arteriosclerotic or multi-infarct)
      dementias   37–38
Vertebro-basilar ischaemia   107
Vertigo   43, 45, 46
Vestibular apparatus   45
Vestibular neuronitis   46
Visual disorders   6, 44, 45, 67–76, 129
   episodic   68–70
   perception   75–76
   persistent and progressive   71–72
Visual hallucinations   75–76
Visuo-spatial disorientation   30
Vitamin B deficiency   109–110, 138
Vitamin B_{12} deficiency   48, 138–139

Walking   9, 43–50
Wasserman reaction   51
Water depletion   80, 132–133
Water intoxication   132
Wernicke's encephalopathy   74, 109–110, 135,
      136
Working diagnosis   13
Writer's cramp   124
Writing   30, 91

X-ray examination   113, 119

Zimmer frame   52, 119